Integrating Quality and Strategy

in Health Care Organizations

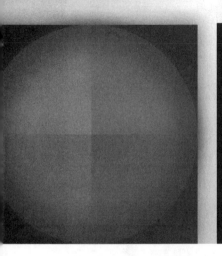

Sarmad Sadeghi, MD, PhD
Taussig Cancer Institute
Cleveland Clinic Foundation
Cleveland, Ohio

Afsaneh Barzi, MD, PhD
Keck Medical Center
Norris Comprehensive Cancer Center
University of Southern California
Los Angeles, California

Osama Mikhail, PhD
Fleming Center for Healthcare Management
School of Public Health
University of Texas Health Science Center at Houston
Houston, Texas

M. Michael Shabot, MD
Memorial Hermann Healthcare System
School of Biomedical Informatics
University of Texas Health Science Center at Houston
Houston, Texas

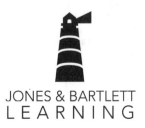

JONES & BARTLETT
LEARNING

World Headquarters
Jones & Bartlett Learning
5 Wall Street
Burlington, MA 01803
978-443-5000
info@jblearning.com
www.jblearning.com

Jones & Bartlett Learning books and products are available through most bookstores and online book-sellers. To contact Jones & Bartlett Learning directly, call 800-832-0034, fax 978-443-8000, or visit our website, www.jblearning.com.

Production Credits
Publisher: Michael Brown
Managing Editor: Maro Gartside
Editorial Assistant: Chloe Falivene
Production Manager: Tracey McCrea
Production Assistant: Alyssa Lawrence
Senior Marketing Manager: Sophie Fleck Teague
Manufacturing and Inventory Control Supervisor: Amy Bacus
Composition: Laserwords Private Limited, Chennai, India
Cover Design: Kristin E. Parker
Cover Image: © Kristin E. Parker
Printing and Binding: Edwards Brothers Malloy
Cover Printing: Edwards Brothers Malloy

Library of Congress Cataloging-in-Publication Data
Integrating quality and strategy in health care organizations / Sarmad Sadeghi ... [et al.].
    p. ; cm.
  Includes bibliographical references and index.
  ISBN 978-0-7637-9540-5 (pbk.)—ISBN 0-7637-9540-2 (pbk.)
  I. Sadeghi, Sarmad.
  [DNLM: 1. Quality Assurance, Health Care—United States. 2. Delivery of Health Care—United States. 3. Health Services—United States. W 84.4 AA1]
  362.1—dc23
                                                              2012008216
6048

Printed in the United States of America
16 15 14 13 12   10 9 8 7 6 5 4 3 2 1

Contents

Foreword

Quality is elusive. Not only achieving it. But defining it. Measuring it. Planning it. And improving it. That's why *Integrating Quality and Strategy in Health Care Organizations* is a book whose time has come. Drs. Sarmad Sadeghi, Afsaneh Barzi, Osama Mikhail, and Michael Shabot take nothing for granted. They provide a bedrock definition for quality. They construct their arguments and observations on a foundational understanding of healthcare organization and the strategic role of quality in the evolving dynamics of the American healthcare system. The result is a document of surpassing utility, combining a basic introduction to the topic of quality in health care with high-level analysis and advice for current and future leaders in medicine and public health.

Quality in health care has moved to the forefront of the national discussion in recent years. Quality and safety are rightfully seen as key to controlling costs and improving outcomes and experience. Healthcare leadership is coming to understand that quality is more than compliance. It needs to become a permanent part of the organizational culture. Moreover, we have to plan to maintain and improve quality going forward. Quality needs to be front and center as we hire, build, and organize for the future. This calls for vision, and a relentless focus on patients and their needs.

I'm pleased to note that the authors of *Integrating Quality and Strategy in Health Care Organizations* include examples from the Cleveland Clinic among their case studies. The Cleveland Clinic pioneered many aspects of quality improvement over the past 30 years. We have been measuring and analyzing volumes, mortality, and other data at increasing levels of magnification. The results include a steady improvement in some key outcomes indicators and a dramatic improvement in others. The Cleveland Clinic's quality improvement efforts have been inestimably aided by two factors. One is the group practice model of medicine, which enables us to implement quality and safety protocols with a minimum of organizational friction. The second is health information technology. We have quality, experience, and utilization dashboards that enable us to gather, visualize, and act on quality data almost instantaneously. These are outstanding tools.

The quality revolution requires aggressive leadership at all levels. Tomorrow's health care will be driven by outcomes, innovation, and service. Those who can build quality into their strategic planning will enjoy the greatest rewards. Not the least of those rewards will be the health of our patients, the safety of our hospitals, and the wellness of our communities.

I would like to thank the authors of *Integrating Quality and Strategy in Health Care Organizations* for their thorough and incisive overview of this all-important topic.

Delos M. Cosgrove, MD
CEO and President of the Cleveland Clinic

Preface

Healthcare organizations are increasingly under financial and regulatory pressures to improve the quality of care they deliver. Public reporting on quality of care is making potential deficiencies visible, which adds to this pressure. In this environment, healthcare organizations are working aggressively to respond to these forces by improving their performance in measures that are under increasing scrutiny.

Unfortunately, only a small, albeit important, portion of the quality challenges is addressed in this fashion. There are several causes for this, but perhaps the most important ones are the lack of a formal definition and appreciation of quality in its full breadth and depth, and the inability to fully integrate quality into the strategic planning process for healthcare organizations.

This book attempts to fill this gap. It is designed for audiences in classrooms at schools of public health and healthcare administration, as well as executives and managers in healthcare organizations. The authors have tried to present a thorough yet concise review of the current healthcare environment, the history of quality in general, and quality issues specific to the healthcare industry. This is followed by a definition of quality from the Institute of Medicine—which will be repeated as needed throughout the book—and a review of the challenges to quality measurement and the major organizations that provide guidance to healthcare organizations in the management of quality.

Fully integrating quality into the strategic planning process requires a sophisticated quality measurement and monitoring system. The authors present a framework that addresses all of the domains and dimensions of quality and their integration into the range of operational activities within the healthcare organization. A structured approach for reporting quality performance at each operational level along a particular domain or dimension of quality is provided and can be aggregated to multiple levels of the organization. This framework is simple and flexible, yet it allows for straightforward expansion such that every quality related measure for any healthcare operation can be incorporated. The parallels between financial performance and quality performance management are presented and the case is made that ultimately quality performance must reflect the same level of priority and attention as financial performance at both the executive and governance levels. The framework proposed and presented in this book will serve that end.

The landscape of quality performance management in health care is constantly evolving, making it virtually impossible to be current on all aspects related to the subject. However, the authors believe that the framework and principles presented will continue to apply even as some of the specifics evolve. Consequently, the authors remain hopeful that this book will continue to provide a structured basis for dealing with the complex and ever-changing world of quality performance management in healthcare organizations.

Contributors to Chapter 10

Kamyar Afshar, DO
Assistant Professor of Medicine
University of Southern California
Los Angeles, CA

Kevin W. Anderson, MBA
Senior Process Improvement Specialist
Cleveland Clinic
Cleveland, OH

Guido Bergomi
Director of Quality Improvement
Cleveland Clinic
Cleveland, OH

Tammy Campos, RN, MSN
Clinical Director of Patient Care
    MICU, MIMU, RRT
Memorial Hermann Hospital
Texas Medical Center
Houston, TX

Yashwant Chathampally, MD
Assistant Professor of Emergency
    Medical Services–Clinical
Memorial Hermann Hospital
Texas Medical Center
Houston, TX

John Cicero
Director of Clinical Sourcing
Cleveland Clinic
Cleveland, OH

Kathleen Coe, RN, BSN
Keck Medical Center
University of Southern California
Los Angeles, CA

Pratik Doshi, MD
Assistant Professor of Emergency
    Medical Services–Clinical
University of Texas–Houston
Houston, TX

Scott M. Dwyer, MBA
Item Master Manager
Cleveland Clinic
Cleveland, OH

Lynne Gervasi, MSN, MPA
Assistant Director of Patient Safety
Cleveland Clinic
Cleveland, OH

Kathy Hartman, RN, MSN
Senior Director of Health
    Information Management
Cleveland Clinic Health System
Cleveland, OH

J. Michael Henderson, MBChB, FRCS
Chief Quality Officer
Cleveland Clinic Health System
Cleveland, OH

Daniel Hudson, RN, BSN
Keck Medical Center
University of Southern California
Los Angeles, CA

Janice Hughes, RN
Clinical Director of the Emergency
    Center
Memorial Hermann Hospital
Texas Medical Center
Houston, TX

Lillian S. Kao, MD
Associate Professor of Surgery
Memorial Hermann Hospital
Texas Medical Center
Houston, TX

Rachna Priya Khatri, MPH, MBA
Clinical Quality Improvement and
    Planning Manager
University of Texas
Houston Medical School
Houston, TX

Brent King, MD
Clive, Nancy, and Pierce Runnells
    Distinguished Professor of
    Emergency Medicine
Chairman, Department of Emergency
    Medicine
Executive Vice–Dean for Clinical
    Affairs
University of Texas
Houston Medical School
Houston, TX

Dominique LaRochelle, MHA
Project Manager for Quality
    Improvement
Cleveland Clinic
Cleveland, OH

Katharine Luther, RN, MPM
Vice President
Institute for Healthcare Improvement
Cambridge, MA

James J. McCarthy, MD
Assistant Professor of Emergency
    Medical Services–Clinical
Memorial Hermann Hospital
Texas Medical Center
Houston, TX

William Pack
Chief Financial Officer
Memorial Hermann Hospital
Texas Medical Center
Houston, TX

Bela Patel, MD
Associate Professor
Assistant Dean of Healthcare Quality
Division Director of Critical Care
  Medicine
Assistant Chief Medical Officer
Memorial Hermann Hospital
Texas Medical Center
Houston, TX

Robert Patrick, MD, MBA
Hospitalist
Cleveland Clinic
Cleveland, OH

Shannon Connor Phillips, MD, MPH
Quality and Patient Safety Officer
Cleveland Clinic
Cleveland, OH

Sylvia Reimer, RN, LP, CE
Emergency Department
Memorial Hermann Hospital
Texas Medical Center
Houston, TX

Melissa Schlechte
Project Manager for Quality
  Improvement
Cleveland Clinic
Cleveland, OH

Ruth M. Siska, RN
Clinical Nurse Manager
Memorial Hermann Hospital
Texas Medical Center
Houston, TX

Yin Tchen, RN, MHA, JD
Keck Medical Center
University of Southern California
Los Angeles, CA

Anthony J. Warmuth, MPA, FACHE, CPHQ
Administrator of Quality and Patient
  Safety
Cleveland Clinic
Cleveland, OH

Acknowledgments

The authors would like to acknowledge the contributions of James Langabeer who reviewed the early draft, Jennifer Mikhail who did some of the early proof reading, Noel Pugh who made a contribution to our understanding of healthcare reform, Rachna Priya Khatri who has been indispensable in developing some of the cases and organizing some of the chapters, and Janki Panchal who has been diligent in pursuing all of the required copyright permissions.

Introduction

Quality has been an area of fashionable attention in health care for some time; however, recently the focus has begun to shift toward quality as a major (but not sole) concern within the overall context of healthcare reform. For decades, quality was taken for granted, even though neither a clear definition nor expectations of quality care were available. This was challenged by an Institute of Medicine (IOM) report in 2000, *To Err is Human*, which unraveled the entire tapestry of the "best healthcare system in the world."[1] According to IOM's report, up to 98,000 deaths per year were the result of preventable medical errors[1]—a very grim statistic. Suddenly, not only could one not be certain of the quality of care delivered, but also the safety of the care delivered was in question. The "first, do no harm" covenant of medicine was at risk.

In addressing the issue of healthcare quality, the IOM advanced a definition of quality as follows[2,3]:

> The degree to which health services for individuals and populations increase the likelihood of desired health outcomes and are consistent with current professional knowledge.

On the basis of this definition, IOM put forth six aims for the 21st century healthcare system; these aims were intended to make the healthcare system safer, more effective, patient centered, timely, efficient, and equitable.[3]

This was a beginning. Ten years later, many government, private nonprofit, and for-profit organizations entered the arena to help improve the quality of the healthcare system by introducing quality measurement schemes, hospital quality surveys and reports, and so forth. Unfortunately, these efforts have not been well coordinated, and at times have been overlapping, repetitive, and somewhat selective, focusing only on a few aims introduced by IOM and addressing only a limited number of medical conditions. Moreover, the reports and performance measurement systems that have been developed are highly vulnerable to subjective interpretation, can somewhat easily be manipulated and may therefore be misleading, and are not sufficiently comprehensive to be the basis for any decision making, specific or general, by consumers or payers/policy makers, respectively.

Health care has been transformed from individual physicians engaged in medical practice based on their own beliefs and with minimum financial expectations to large, complex enterprises interacting in the delivery of care for an individual. As best stated by Paul Starr in *The Social Transformation of American Medicine*, medicine has gone from a "sovereign profession to a vast industry."[4]

Quality was, is, and always will be expected from healthcare organizations. What is changing is the shift from a general "trust" of physicians and other healthcare professionals to a skepticism that now demands scientific measurement and transparency—basically a shift away from acceptance of the "art" of medicine to reliance on the "science" of medicine (to the extent that it exists). Whereas trust might have been the only basis for quality expectations in the context of one individual physician–patient interaction, more measures of quality are needed for a multi-tier interaction in the complex healthcare system of today.[5] The quality measurement movement removes a reliance solely on professionalism and focuses on other means to measure (and ensure) quality.

Expansion of managed care in health care is another reason for growing concerns over quality. Managed care organizations have financial liabilities and the interest of their shareholders in addition to the interest of their enrollees, which can create conflicts of interest.[6]

Several other factors make healthcare quality a very important topic. The first of these factors is cost considerations. As it is well known, the societal cost of health care is rising rapidly, and at the same time the government is trying to contain cost while maintaining or even improving quality.[7] In fact, cost is a very important consideration in the quality movement in health care.[8] Historically, quality in manufacturing was reformed under the pressure of resource limitations and cost containment. Similarly, the rising cost of health care and pressure from consumers, the government, and managed care organizations are the drivers of the quality movement in health care.

Shortfalls in quality include overuse, underuse, and misuse of the services.[9,10] Decrease of overuse and prevention of misuse will decrease the cost of health care; however, decrease of underuse will increase the overall cost of health care in the short run, but might prove to be a cost-saving investment decades later.

All of these factors have made attention to quality in health care a necessity; awareness of the high rate of *defects* in current practices in health care has been sobering. The thought of having similar defect rates in other industries could not be more frightening. At a defect rate of 20%, which is reported to happen in the use of antibiotics for colds, there would be 9 million daily errors in credit card transactions, 36 million checks would be deposited in the wrong accounts every day, and there would be a 1,000-fold increase in deaths from airplane crashes.[11]

There is no question that quality must improve. Regulatory initiatives influenced by the requirements of accrediting organizations such as The Joint Commission (TJC) and Det Norske Veritas (DNV) have been successful but are by no means comprehensive or sufficient. There must be a multilateral effort by all parties involved including consumers and regulatory bodies, not just the providers and payers, to create a will that is strong enough to move this $2.6 trillion[12] industry toward reducing the rate of preventable defects to a level comparable with that of other industries while at the same time creating an environment that provides care that is comparable across dimensions of geography and socioeconomic status. Goals must be set high; only then can there be consistent and evidence-based care delivered to all. And only then can there be hope to be rid of staggering nonproductive costs such as malpractice insurance and defensive medicine.

Medical care is delivered in a complex environment that is in desperate need of reform. The first step would be the recognition that the United States population does not have the best health in the world.[13]

In a discussion about quality in health care, one would hear, most frequently, about quality improvement *initiatives* and quality-enhancing *projects*, or *tactics* to improve quality in the context of a healthcare organization. For this text, the principal healthcare organization is the hospital, and it therefore represents the primary healthcare setting for the text. These tactics for improvement of quality should be integrated into an organization's strategy and may well represent a significant portion of that organization's strategic plan or multiyear programs. The goal is often to satisfy regulatory requirements, or enhance the organization's standing with an accrediting organization or Medicare or, although less frequently, maintain or improve the organization's standing on the *U.S. News & World Report* ranking.

Furthermore, when quality is looked at in terms of an initiative, project, or tactical move, the impact of other parts of the organization's strategic or multiyear plan is rarely factored in the final outcome. It is conceivable that other competing initiatives may undermine the quality initiative. As an example, one could think of two initiatives: a cost-containment project that reduces staff in a lab, which may affect error rates, and an addition of new equipment for greater accuracy in lab results—the net effect on quality may be unpredictable.

Therefore, management may consider that any and all initiatives in a strategic plan may have direct, indirect, or even unintended positive or negative impact on the quality of care delivered in its organization. As a result, management should evaluate the impact of any strategic plan on the quality of the organization's products or services before entering the execution phase. Furthermore, the impact on quality should be regarded as a critical consideration in determining the overall advisability of the plan.

This brings up the following question: What is the appropriate placement of quality and quality performance in the context of an organization's priorities and strategic direction? This is followed by the question: How can quality considerations be integrated into the strategy development process so that a variety of consumer, payer, competitive, and regulatory concerns are addressed adequately and in a systematic fashion? The answers to these questions and others embody the contribution of this text to the management literature and are further discussed in the chapters.

HOW TO USE THIS BOOK

This text is divided into 10 chapters. Although the discussion starts with quality as a general concept and then transitions from a history of the quality movement in manufacturing to the modern healthcare system, the frameworks offered and discussed here focus on the quality of health care delivered in the inpatient setting of a hospital organization. It is, however, possible to expand these frameworks to apply to other contexts, such as organizations that focus mainly on outpatient care delivery or organizations that provide care in both inpatient and outpatient settings.

Chapter 1: Understanding the U.S. Healthcare System

Chapter 1 aims to set the stage for the topics covered in this book. A healthcare organization is part of a very complex industry with many moving parts that interact with each other and also with the environment. To understand the organization and to contemplate organizational strategy requires an understanding of the industry and its environment. To that end, a brief historical review of the U.S. healthcare system and its evolution seems to be the appropriate overture to the primary topic of this text. In this chapter, the forces that impinge on a healthcare organization are identified and discussed. This chapter was written during a major regulatory overhaul of the healthcare system by the Obama administration, and therefore it is important and necessary to address the impact of reform on quality. As such, the authors will seek answers to the following questions in an objective manner:

1. What characterizes the U.S. healthcare system today?
2. What are the highlights of historical healthcare reform movements?
3. What are the major elements of the reform and how will they impact the healthcare system?

Chapter 2: Understanding the Healthcare Organization

Chapter 2 addresses the general management structure of a healthcare organization. This organizational structure is responsible for developing the strategic plan that establishes priorities and direction for the healthcare organization. Depending on the specific healthcare focus and size of the organization, its management structure can vary. However, to perform well in the U.S. healthcare environment, there is a set of managerial and governance functions that every organization must incorporate and execute reasonably well.

Chapter 2 will seek to answer the following questions:

1. What are the typical management structures and the corresponding scopes of responsibilities?
2. What is a typical strategic planning process like?
3. What is the relationship between strategic planning, strategy execution, and operational activities within the organization?

Chapter 3: General Concepts in Quality

Chapter 3 aims to understand the evolution of quality from a historical perspective with an initial look at manufacturing where many of the principles of quality assurance and improvement were developed. From there, differences between manufacturing and healthcare industries will be pointed out to create a better understanding of which concepts and principles from manufacturing may be readily adopted and which may need to be adjusted or set aside. This is followed by a review of the literature dealing with quality of inpatient care and concludes by presenting a widely accepted definition for healthcare quality that will form the basis for a more detailed and more operational approach to measuring, managing, and improving the quality of inpatient care.

In Chapter 3, the following specific questions are discussed:

1. How is quality addressed in other industries, and what impact has this had on addressing quality in health care?
2. What is healthcare quality, and what are the similarities and differences between it and manufacturing or service quality.
3. What is an operational framework for and definition of healthcare quality?

Chapter 4: Current State of Quality Measurement: External Dynamics

Chapter 4 aims to show the current state of healthcare quality measurement. To that end, a representative group of organizations that are active in the field of healthcare quality will be reviewed. A summary that captures each organization's contribution to the field of healthcare quality will be presented.

In Chapter 4, the following specific questions are discussed:

1. What are the active organizations in various healthcare quality-related areas?
2. What are the primary functions of these organizations and what stake-holders are represented by them?

Chapter 5: Current State of Quality Measurement: Internal Dynamics

The objective of Chapter 5 is to give a brief overview of some of the concepts, stakeholders, and dynamics of managing the quality of care that is delivered by a healthcare organization. The most important quality measures, proposed by the organizations discussed in Chapter 4, have made it to the radar screens of most healthcare organizations, and monitors and controls have been set up not only to have information about the status of those measures, but also to be able to respond to deficiencies and provide mechanisms for course correction.

Healthcare organizations, in adapting to external forces, have developed methods to automate and streamline their control over the quality measures. This chapter attempts to answer the following questions:

1. What is involved in establishing a culture of quality within a healthcare organization?
2. How has safety become synonymous with quality?
3. Do these efforts sufficiently address the quality needs of the modern healthcare organization?

Chapter 6: Measuring Quality of Inpatient Care

The objective of Chapter 6 is to present a framework for the measurement of (inpatient) healthcare quality, as defined in Chapter 3. This framework is intended to provide a basis for inpatient healthcare providers operationally to define, measure, report, and improve quality of care in a way that can meaning-fully be addressed at multiple levels within the provider organization. The supporting literature and logical backbone of this framework is also discussed. The following questions are specifically discussed:

1. What would a quality measurement system that is consistent with IOM aims look like?
2. How can such a system be made operational and geared toward a specific organization?
3. How can measures across domains and dimensions of quality be aggre-gated in a logical fashion to create broader reports of an organization's performance?

Chapter 7: Understanding Quality and Performance

The aim of Chapter 7 is to develop a deeper understanding of the quality of medical care in a healthcare organization. This is followed by an effort to answer the following specific questions:

1. What are the interactions between strategy, organizational performance, finance, and quality?
2. Who is accountable for the quality of care delivered by an organization?
3. What is value in health care?
4. How are strategic decisions made? How should they be made?

After a discussion of what is involved in formulating a strategy and the sig-nificance and importance of quality in this process, the stage is set for Chapter 8.

Chapter 8: Quantifying the Quality Performance Gaps

The objective of Chapter 8 is to lay out a strategy development framework driven by organizational performance considerations. This framework is based on the setting of performance targets and then identification of gaps between the current status and the performance targets. In contrast to the conventional finance-centered planning process, this framework will require an estimation of not only financial consequences but also quality consequences of any strategy considered by the organization. In such a context, the following questions need to be answered:

1. How can quality measures be identified and used in this framework?
2. How should the targets be set and the gaps measured?

Once performance gaps are measured, the organization is ready to develop a strategic plan to achieve the performance targets within a specified time frame. This will be discussed in Chapter 9.

Chapter 9: Closing the Gaps

The objective of Chapter 9 is to develop this framework further and include control mechanisms for strategy selection and course corrections during implementation. Here the following questions will be addressed:

1. How can various strategies be described with respect to healthcare quality?
2. How should quality performance be monitored and course correction implemented in the organization?

Chapter 10: Case Studies in Healthcare Quality

Chapter 10 will provide a series of healthcare quality improvement case studies from different institutions. Each case study illustrates a systematic approach to a quality problem.

REFERENCES

1. Kohn LCJ, Donaldson M. *To Err is Human: Building a Safer Health System.* Washington, DC: National Academy Press; 2000.
2. Lohr KN. *Medicare: A Strategy for Quality Assurance.* Vol 1. Washington, DC: Institute of Medicine; 1990.
3. Committee on Quality of Health Care in America. *Crossing the Quality Chasm: A New Health System for the 21st Century.* Washington, DC: Institute of Medicine; 2001.
4. Starr P. *The Social Transformation of American Medicine.* New York, NY: Basic Books; 1982.
5. Shortell SM, Waters TM, Clarke KW, Budetti PP. Physicians as double agents: maintaining trust in an era of multiple accountabilities. *JAMA.* 1998;280(12):1102–1108.
6. Angell M, Kassirer JP. Quality and the medical marketplace—following elephants. *N Engl J Med.* 1996;335(12):883–885.
7. Blumenthal D. Quality of health care. Part 4: the origins of the quality-of-care debate. *N Engl J Med.* 1996;335(15):1146–1149.
8. Orszag P. *The Overuse, Underuse and Misuse of Health Care.* Washington, DC: Congressional Budget Office; 2008.

9. Donaldson MS. *Measuring the Quality of Health Care*. Washington, DC: Institute of Medicine; 1999.

10. Chassin MR, Galvin RW, National Roundtable on Health Care Quality. The urgent need to improve health care quality: Institute of Medicine National Roundtable on Health Care Quality. *JAMA.* 1998;280(11):1000–1005.

11. Chassin MR. Is health care ready for Six Sigma quality? *Milbank Q.* 1998;76(4): 565–591, 510.

12. U.S. Department of Health and Human Services. *National Health Expenditure Projections 2007–2017.* Washington, DC: Department of Health and Human Services; 2007.

13. Starfield B. Is US health really the best in the world? *JAMA.* 2000;284(4):483–485.

Understanding the U.S. Healthcare System

INTRODUCTION

The long-term success and prosperity of an organization is inextricably linked to the strategy it pursues over time. A firm understanding of the environment within which the organization exists is a critical ingredient in the strategy development process. This chapter identifies both the stakeholders in the healthcare system and the environmental forces that are at work and must be taken into account in the formulation of strategy.

The dramatic growth in the size and cost of the U.S. healthcare industry in the past few decades has refocused all stakeholders (providers, suppliers, payers, and consumers) on one message: the current trend is not sustainable. In response to this, stakeholders (perhaps excluding consumers) have pursued strategies that would enhance their individual positions in this sector of the economy. Fortunately, it would seem that most of these strategies have at their core a common concept: value (i.e., benefit versus cost) derived from health services provided, consumed, and reimbursed. Analyzing these forces with respect to the value proposition provides guidance to the organization's management with respect to setting of priorities, allocation of resources, and development of strategy.

In March 2010, in a rare and historic move, the U.S. Congress passed the Patient Protection and Affordable Care Act (PPACA), which was signed into law by President Obama and created significant changes that impact virtually every healthcare organization. Access and value (as defined by quality of care relative to the cost of care) are recurring themes in the legislation and will be discussed later in this text as both are directly related to quality. The changes as a result of this legislation permeate the industry and will have a significant impact on payers and providers. Therefore, some of the more prominent components of these changes are discussed in this chapter.

GOALS AND OBJECTIVES

This chapter is designed to help the reader develop a firm grasp of the various components of the U.S. healthcare system and understand the major issues faced by the stakeholders within the system. Along with the next chapter, it serves as a foundation for the strategy development discussions presented later in this text.

After reading this chapter, the reader should be able to:

1. Categorize and describe the stakeholders in the U.S. healthcare system.
2. Discuss the performance of the U.S. healthcare system.
3. Discuss the differences in performance between the U.S. healthcare system and an average healthcare system in the industrialized world.
4. Discuss the major issues faced by the U.S. healthcare system.
5. Discuss the rising costs of care and its major components.
6. Discuss the problem of access and lack of universal healthcare coverage in the United States.
7. Discuss the highlights of the history of healthcare reform in the United States.
8. Discuss how reforms have addressed some of the performance challenges of the U.S. healthcare system.

THE U.S. HEALTHCARE SYSTEM STRUCTURE

The U.S. healthcare system is a product of decades of growth and maturation that too often have led to a variety of deficiencies and serious problems. The responses to these problems, whether they came from the private sector or the government, have frequently been only short-term corrections. This shortsightedness in addressing the healthcare system's problems is a product of the preoccupation of most businesses with short-term financial performance at the expense of thoughtful and responsible course correction and the preoccupation of politicians with political gamesmanship and elections. As a result, the system is a complex of layered adjustments made up mostly of patchwork and temporary fixes to such an extent that any intelligent design is undetectable. This short-term thinking and the unintended consequences of legislated policies have created a complex healthcare system that is inefficient and difficult to understand.

At the core of any healthcare system, including the U.S. healthcare system, a product or service is offered to a consumer at a certain price. The rules that govern such transactions come from various entities, but all are expected to comply with the laws of their country—in this case, the United States. As such, one can categorize the major stakeholders as regulators and policy makers, payers, advocacy organizations, providers, suppliers, and consumers. These are broad categories that at times overlap, such that one entity may have more than one role; for example, a consumer may also be the payer. These will be discussed in more detail in the paragraphs that follow.

Regulators and Policy Makers in the U.S. Healthcare System

At the top of the pyramid, the federal government sets the tone for the entire system. Many other entities have been formed over the years in response to the need for control over various areas of the healthcare industry. Today, the most influential regulators include the U.S. Department of Health and Human Services (HHS), the Centers for Medicare & Medicaid Services (CMS), the Food and Drug Administration (FDA), and the Centers for Disease Control and Prevention (CDC). These entities have been charged to interpret, implement, and ensure compliance with the current laws of the United States that affect and govern the healthcare industry. The scope of regulatory influence of these entities is determined by the laws they enforce.

At the state level, state legislatures, state and local governments, health departments, state medical boards, and state insurance commissions also play significant roles while functioning within federal regulations. Nevertheless, state governments have been successful in introducing unprecedented moves that go beyond federal mandates for healthcare policy; for example, Massachusetts was able to mandate health insurance coverage for all its citizens in 2006.[1]

Payers in the U.S. Healthcare System

Financing in the U.S. healthcare system can be broken down into payments made by the public sector (the federal government, state and local governments), the private sector (private insurers and businesses), and the consumer (out-of-pocket expenses and self-pay). The share of each source in the total national healthcare expenditure in 2008 is shown in **Figure 1-1**.

As can be seen in the chart, 47% of the expenditure comes from public sources and 53% from private sources. Public funding of the U.S. healthcare system includes federal sources, such as Medicare and Medicaid programs, the Veterans Administration, and the U.S. Department of Defense, and state and local programs, such as Medicaid and state and local hospitals. Private funding includes out-of-pocket expenditure, private insurance, and philanthropy. As can be inferred from this list, many of these payers have other capacities and exert substantial influence in other areas of the U.S. healthcare system through policy making (e.g., CMS) or through advocacy groups and lobbying (e.g., private insurance companies).

Advocacy Organizations

This category encompasses organized efforts of smaller entities in the healthcare system around a common interest that is frequently self-serving. These organizations are numerous, and discussion of their role and influence in the U.S.

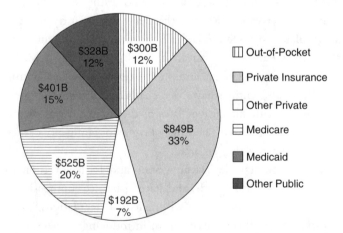

FIGURE 1-1. In 2010, the total national healthcare expenditure was $2,594 billion. The breakdown of where this money came from is presented in this chart. B, billion. Data from CMS.[2]

healthcare system is beyond the scope of this text. Examples of these groups include the American Medical Association (AMA), the American Society of Clinical Oncology (ASCO), the American Hospital Association (AHA), the American Nurses Association (ANA), America's Health Insurance Plans (AHIP), and the National Patient Advocate Foundation (NPAF).

Providers in the U.S. Healthcare System

This category includes all individuals and organizations that provide a healthcare service to the consumer. As such, it includes health practitioners, hospitals, nursing homes, and other similar entities. Although health professionals are central to the specific entity that actually provides care, hospitals, in particular, offer the environment in which care can be provided and are compensated by payers for the services provided. It is in the hospital setting that a substantial portion of healthcare resources are consumed.

Individual practitioners, practice groups, general hospitals, specialty hospitals, ambulatory facilities (surgery, imaging, etc.), and integrated healthcare systems are also examples of providers.

Suppliers

This category includes pharmaceutical companies and medical equipment companies. These entities have grown to be a significant part of the healthcare system and are in fact considered industries of their own. Although suppliers are integral to the healthcare system, the nature of their business is different. Like private insurance companies, most of these organizations are for-profit and publicly traded companies and exist in a different competitive environment. Unlike the payer category, the amount of not-for-profit activity in this category is small.

Consumers

People, whether sick or healthy, are consumers of care. In the industrialized world, one would be hard pressed to find anyone who has never received any care within a healthcare system. Consumers of healthcare services are somewhat different from consumers in other sectors of the economy. Two primary differences are (1) healthcare consumers often have to depend on the advice of a physician in making a health services "consumption" decision, and (2) in most instances, the consumer is unaware of the full costs of his or her choice because of the intermediary function of payers—even though there may be a significant out-of-pocket component of the full cost.

THE U.S. HEALTHCARE SYSTEM PERFORMANCE

From a global systems perspective, the performance of a healthcare system can be viewed in terms of the size and makeup of the population it serves, the healthcare outcomes it produces, and the amount of resources it consumes. Other factors, such as fairness issues that include equitable distribution of the healthcare services and financial burden and quality of care delivered within the system, should also be included in the mix.

The World Health Organization (WHO) proposed a framework for measurement of performance at the level of a healthcare system by first defining healthcare action as "any set of activities whose primary intent is to improve or maintain health."[3] This definition establishes boundaries within which the framework measures performance around three fundamental goals: improving health, enhancing responsiveness to the expectations of the population, and ensuring fairness of financial contribution.

Improvement of health involves both increase of average health status and decrease of health inequalities. Responsiveness involves respect for the individual (i.e., dignity, confidentiality, and autonomy) and client orientation (e.g., prompt attention and choice of provider). Fairness of financial contribution implies that the individual is protected from financial risks due to health care.

Based on this framework, performance relates attainment of the aforementioned goals to the resource allocation; furthermore, variations in performance are the results of four key functions: (1) stewardship (broader than regulation only), (2) financing, (3) service provision, and (4) resource generation. WHO suggests that by investigating these four functions, it is possible to understand the determinants of health system performance and identify major policy challenges.[3]

This framework was also adopted by the Organisation for Economic Co-operation and Development (OECD) with slight modification. In this modified framework, access to health care and outcomes are included among the goals (**Table 1-1**).

Table 1-1 Health System Goals in Relation to the Component for Assessment[4]

	Average Level	Distribution
Health Improvement/Outcomes (+)	✓	✓
Responsiveness and Access (+)	✓	✓
Financial Contribution/Health Expenditure (−)	✓	✓
	Efficiency	Equity

As seen in Table 1-1, this framework also links efficiency and equity to the performance measurement process. This framework sets three goals: higher levels of health improvement/outcomes, higher levels of responsiveness and access, and lower levels of financial contribution and health expenditures subject to the successful attainment of the first two goals.[4]

In the following sections, a current status of each of the three main goals in the U.S. healthcare system will be presented from a societal point of view.

Outcomes in the U.S. Healthcare System

Comparing the U.S. data with that of other countries could substantially contribute to one's understanding of what is right and what is not right in the U.S. healthcare system. To that end, a few key pieces of data are presented here.

As will be discussed later in this chapter, the United States is the only industrialized country in the world that does not offer universal healthcare coverage to its citizens. Infant mortality rate has steadily declined in industrialized countries over the past decades, but for the first time since records have been kept, the U.S. rate for infant mortality has climbed above that of the OECD median (**Figure 1-2**).[5]

Potential years of life lost due to diabetes per 100,000 population for the United States is 99, almost 3 times as high as the OECD median, and life expectancy at birth for the United States was 1.3 years lower than the OECD median in 2009 (in 1960 it was 1.7 years higher than the OECD median).[6,7] The United States has the second highest rate of hospital admission for asthma among the OECD countries (121 per 100,000, after the Slovak Republic

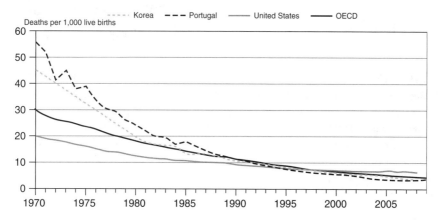

FIGURE 1-2. Data for 2009 from OECD.[5]

with 167 per 100,000), which is more than 2 times the OECD median of 52 per 100,000, whereas Canada and Mexico each have among the lowest rates, 16 and 19 per 100,000, respectively.[8]

The United States spends significantly more than other industrialized nations on health care, both as a percentage of gross domestic product (GDP)[9] and per capita[10] (**Figure 1-3** and **Figure 1-4**). Unfortunately, this spending does not translate into outcomes, for example, life expectancy at birth (**Figure 1-5**).

This suggests that there are significant inefficiencies in the U.S. healthcare system and that the *value** of the services in the U.S. healthcare system may be lower compared with that in other industrialized countries. Discussion of why this may be the case is beyond the scope of this text. However, addressing access to health care in the United States can significantly increase the magnitude of

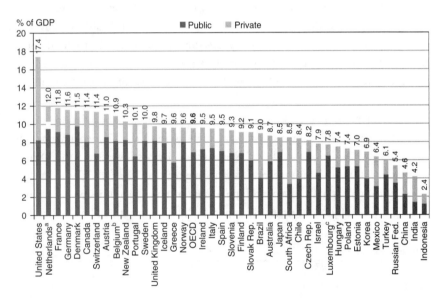

FIGURE 1-3. Total health expenditure as a share of GDP in 2009 (or nearest year). The United States spends more dollars as a percentage of GDP than any other country. [a]In the Netherlands, it is not possible to clearly distinguish the public and private share related to investments. [b]Total expenditure excluding investments. [c]Health expenditure is for the insured population rather than the resident population. From OECD.[9]

---

*Value is proportional to the ratio of quality or outcomes to costs, as discussed in the following chapters.

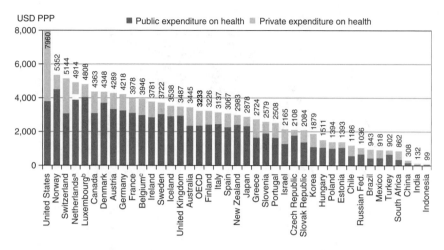

FIGURE 1-4. Total public and private health expenditure per capita in 2009 (or nearest year). The United States spends more dollars per capita than any other country. [a]In the Netherlands, it is not possible to clearly distinguish the public and private share related to investments. [b]Health expenditure is for the insured population rather than the resident population. [c]Total expenditure excluding investments. USD PPP, US$ purchasing power parity. From OECD.[10]

the beneficial effects of primary and preventive care by reducing the uninsured population. This could prevent the expensive complications of chronic conditions such as asthma, chronic obstructive pulmonary disease (COPD), diabetes, hypertension, and atherosclerosis, improving the outcomes for all. This improves quality and creates additional value by way of more equitable access and better outcomes.

Ironically, when compared with the countries that have public healthcare systems, the current healthcare system in the United States, which relies on the efficiency of markets and competition, has the highest administrative cost per capita ($486), twice as much as that for France, which occupies the second place at $243 among the OECD countries.[6]

Access in the U.S. Healthcare System

The U.S. government does not offer universal healthcare coverage to its citizens. As a result, a significant portion of the population does not have health insurance, and to access healthcare services within the system, individuals would have to pay out of pocket. This has been a primary reason for lack of access to health

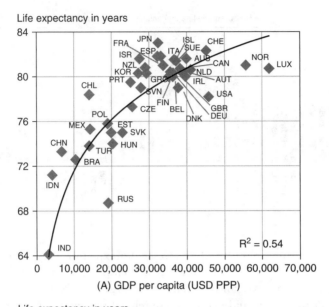

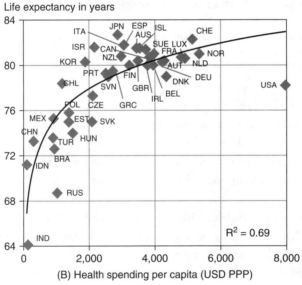

FIGURE 1-5. Correlation between GDP per capita (A), health spending per capita (B), and life expectancy at birth in OECD countries in 2007. The United States is one of the outliers in both curves.[7] USD PPP, US$ purchasing power parity.

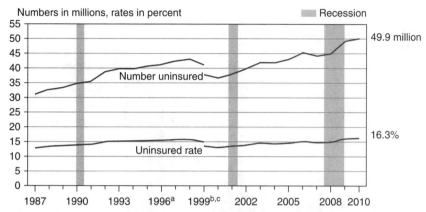

Numbers in millions, rates in percent

Recession

49.9 million

16.3%

a The data for 1996 through 1999 were revised using an approximation method for consistency with the revision to the 2004 and 2005 estimates.
b Implementation of Census 2000–based population controls occurred for the 2000 Annual Social and Economic Supplement (ASEC), which collected data for 1999. These estimates also reflect the results of follow-up verification questions, which were asked of people who responded "no" to all questions about specific types of health insurance coverage in order to verify whether they were actually uninsured. This change increased the number and percentage of people covered by health insurance, bringing the Current Population Survey (CPS) more in line with estimates from other national surveys.
c The data for 1999 through 2009 were revised to reflect the results of enhancements to the editing process.
Note: Respondents were not asked detailed health insurance questions before the 1988 CPS.

FIGURE 1-6. Number of uninsured and the uninsured rate, 1987–2010. The rate of the uninsured has been growing over the years. From DeNavas-Walt et al.[11]

care. Uninsured individuals that are unable to pay often get the care they need through emergency departments when they are very sick, after the opportunity to avoid preventable conditions has long passed.

Unfortunately, the uninsured make up a significant and growing percentage of the U.S. population (**Figure 1-6**). The U.S. Census Bureau estimates the number of uninsured in 2010 at 49.9 million.[11]

As will be discussed later in this chapter, the PPACA, which was signed into law in March 2010, requires most U.S. citizens and legal residents to purchase qualifying health plans or pay a penalty.[12]

Expenditures in the U.S. Healthcare System

In 2010, national healthcare expenditure (NHE) amounted to $2.6 trillion, which is 17.9% of GDP in 2010.[13] For 2012 national healthcare expenditure is

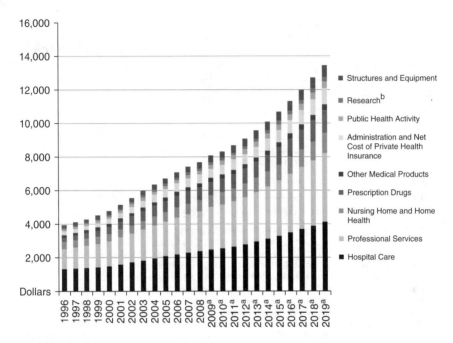

FIGURE 1-7. U.S. healthcare expenditure per capita. [a]Years 2009 through 2019 are based on projections. [b]Research and development expenditures of drug companies and other manufacturers and providers of medical equipment and supplies are excluded from research expenditures. These research expenditures are implicitly included in the expenditure class in which the product falls, in that they are covered by the payment received for that product. Data from U.S. Census Bureau.[14]

projected to go well over $2.8 trillion[15], which is 17.7% of the projected GDP for 2012.[16] **Figure 1-7** illustrates the per capita healthcare expenditures in the United States since 1996.

The national healthcare expenditure as a percentage of GDP has been increasing each year, as seen in **Figure 1-8**. This rate of growth is well above the inflation rate and has proved difficult to control.[2,17] Another concerning trend is that the national healthcare expenditure as a portion of GDP is also growing, essentially at the expense of lack of growth or shrinkage in other sectors (Figure 1-8).

Healthcare expenditures were thought to be immune from economic fluctuations, but the recent economic recession caused a decrease in expenditure growth rate to a historic low of 3.8% in 2009 and 3.9% in 2010, but projections for

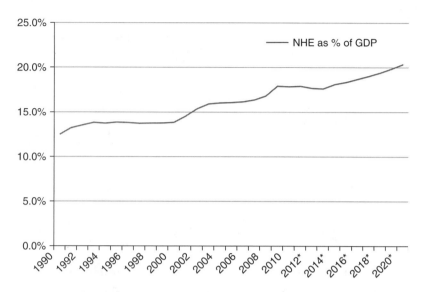

FIGURE 1-8. National healthcare expenditure (NHE) as a percentage of GDP. *Projection. Data from the Congressional Budget Office (CBO)[18] and CMS.[2]

2011 through 2014 show a continued increase in the healthcare expenditure growth rate.[14,16] (**Figure 1-9**).

The breakdown of where this money is spent is shown in **Figure 1-10**. Hospital care and professional services make up more than 60% of the expenditure, followed by prescription drugs.

PERFORMANCE CHALLENGES IN THE U.S. HEALTHCARE SYSTEM

For years, the challenges facing the U.S. healthcare system, including the rising costs and growing number of uninsured individuals, have been the topics of discussion in various business and policy circles. There has been no shortage of prescribed remedies for these challenges, which have ranged from leaving it to the markets, managed care, managed competition, evidence-based medicine, and single-payer universal coverage, none of which are mutually exclusive. To this, one must add growing concerns for the quality of care and increased awareness of poor outcomes within the system.

The response to these challenges can be grouped into two major components: cost containment and improved access. Both of these components play roles in

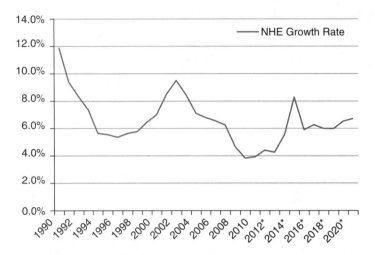

FIGURE 1-9. Growth rate for national healthcare expenditures. National healthcare expenditures have been growing at a rate of more than 5%, with the exception of a temporary dip in years 2008, 2009, and 2010 to 4.4%, 3.8%, and 3.9%, respectively. Mainly attributable to the slump in the U.S. economy.[19–23] *Projection. Data from CMS.[2]

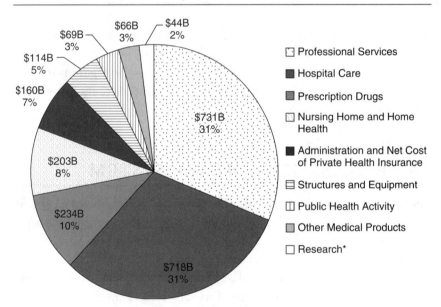

FIGURE 1-10. National healthcare expenditure in 2009: A breakdown of where the money is spent in the U.S. healthcare system. *Research and development expenditures of drug companies and other manufacturers and providers of medical equipment and supplies are excluded as they are implicitly included in the expenditure class in which the product falls. Data from CMS.[2]

the issues associated with healthcare quality measurement and improvement and will be separately discussed.

Healthcare Cost Containment

This has been a topic of great interest over the years, but as shown in the previous sections, healthcare costs continue to rise. To understand how these costs can be controlled, one must understand not only where the money comes from and where it goes, but more importantly what is driving these increases in costs. Typical cost-containment efforts would begin with identifying the major components and drivers of cost and examining opportunities for reductions in those components.

According to the CMS, changes in prices, specifically in medicine, as well as aging and an increase in population account for the majority of the growth of personal healthcare expenditures.[24] As shown in Figure 1-9, professional services, hospital care, and prescription drugs account for more than 70% of the national healthcare expenditure. This is followed by nursing home and administrative costs, which make up another 15% of the costs. This contributes to why chronic disease management, aging of the population, prescription drugs, and administrative costs are among the major factors considered in discussions of costs in health care.[25,26] Whereas one can address some of these drivers, clearly certain factors, such as an aging population, are not controllable.

In addition to age, other demographic factors should also be considered as explanatory but not necessarily controllable factors. Five percent of the U.S. population spends approximately 48% of all healthcare dollars, and 1% of the U.S. population spends more than 20% of the healthcare dollars[27] (**Figure 1-11**).

Geographic variations in healthcare expenditures are also noteworthy in the study of healthcare costs. These differences in costs have been the subject of studies and are not explained by differences in prices alone and may be attributable to utilization.[28,29] These geographical variations are important and controversial[29–32] and are not linked to improved quality[28,33,34] (**Figure 1-12** and **Figure 1-13**).

Another significant problem with healthcare expenditures is the waste in the system defined as "healthcare spending that can be eliminated without reducing the quality of care."[34] This has been a focus of discussion for some time but recently has come under closer scrutiny and is estimated to be upward of $700 billion annually. This is about 30% of the total expenditure and includes unnecessary care (40%), fraud (19%), administrative inefficiency (17%), healthcare provider errors (12%), preventable conditions (6%), and lack of care coordination (6%).[35,36]

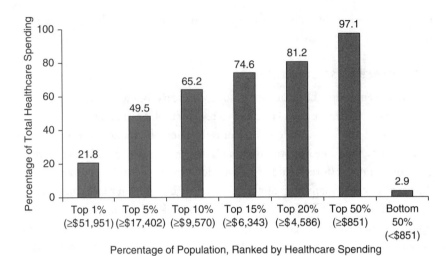

FIGURE 1-11. Concentration of healthcare spending in the U.S. population, 2009. Dollar amounts in parentheses are the annual expenses per person in each percentile. Population is the civilian noninstitutionalized population, including those without any healthcare spending. Healthcare spending is total payments from all sources (including direct payments from individuals, private insurance, Medicare, Medicaid, and miscellaneous other sources) to hospitals, physicians, other providers (including dental care), and pharmacies; health insurance premiums are not included. From Kaiser Family Foundation calculations[27] using data from the U.S. Department of Health and Human Services, Agency for Healthcare Research and Quality, Medical Expenditure Panel Survey (MEPS), 2009.

As can be seen in the data presented thus far, healthcare costs have been rising regardless of the efforts made by the regulators and payers to contain them.[37] Perhaps the most well-known "failed" model has been that of the managed care organizations. Data suggest that managed care organizations were successful in containing costs in the early 1990s by controlling utilization, although this may have come at the expense of quality.[33,38] This practice quickly became equally unpopular among patients and physicians and led to the failure of the managed care model. However, there is empirical evidence that the use of gatekeepers in the managed care model still continues.[38]

A number of approaches have been proposed by experts to bring the costs under some control and include investment in information technology (IT), improvement of quality of care to increase efficiency, adjustment of provider compensation, additional government regulation, preventive medicine, increase in consumer

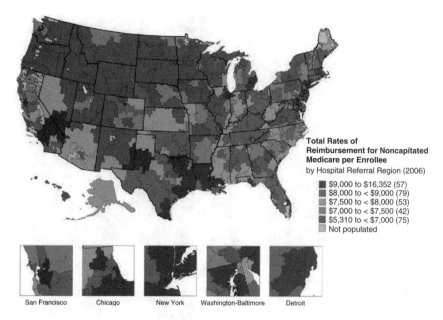

FIGURE 1-12. *Dartmouth Atlas* graphic demonstrating geographical variations in healthcare costs.[34]

involvement and price transparency, and finally tax incentives to expand insurance coverage.[26] To this list one must add reduction of waste in the system as it is a significant proportion of the overall expenditures and merits its own category.[36,39]

Healthcare Access

Decreased access and reduced utilization are sometimes by-products of cost pressures in the industry. Rising costs have resulted in a greater share of the costs being passed on to individuals and families in the form of increased premiums, higher deductibles, and other out-of-pocket expenses—the exclusion of preexisting conditions will also contribute to increased costs.

This problem of increasing costs is unlikely to be solved without the intervention of policy makers and has become a platform for calls for reform. If one day some form of basic healthcare coverage is offered to all of the U.S. population, then the United States will become the last Western country to offer universal coverage. It is important to recognize that the issue of access is not only a matter of fairness, equity, or even quality. Limited access only postpones the need to deal with a medical problem that inevitably comes back in the form of a complicated medical condition in need of urgent or emergent attention. The Emergency

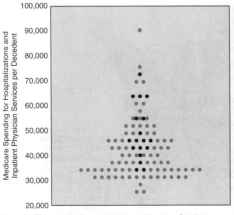

Selected Academic Medical Center Data	
Cedars-Sinai Medical Center	$71,637
UCLA Medical Center	$63,900
Johns Hopkins Hospital	$63,079
New York-Presbyterian Hospital	$62,773
UCSF Medical Center	$54,669
Hospital of the University of Pennsylvania	$54,455
Brigham and Women's Hospital	$50,156
University of Washington Medical Center	$46,891
University of Michigan Hospitals	$46,397
University of Chicago Hospital	$45,718
Stanford Hospital and Clinics	$44,997
UPMC Presbyterian Shadyside	$43,504
Yale-New Haven Hospital	$43,325
Massachusetts General Hospital	$43,058
Barnes-Jewish Hospital	$40,681
Duke University Hospital	$37,751
Cleveland Clinic Foundation	$34,437
Mayo Clinic (St. Mary's Hospital)	$34,372

Medicare Spending for Hospitalizations and Inpatient Physician Services per Decedent in the Last Two Years of Life Among Patients with At Least One of Nine Chronic Conditions Receiving Most of their Care from Selected COTH Integrated Academic Medical Centers (Deaths Occurring 2001–2005)

Among COTH integrated academic medical centers, per decedent Medicare reimbursements for inpatient care during the last two years of life varied by a factor of four, from about $24,000 to almost $92,000. Each point represents one of the 93 selected COTH academic medical centers. The 18 hospitals on USN&WR's Honor Roll for 2007 are highlighted in red.

FIGURE 1-13. Geographical differences in spending illustrated across major medical centers of national and international reputation. Spending at Cedars-Sinai Medical Center is more than two times higher than that at the Mayo Clinic and the Cleveland Clinic.[32]

Medical Treatment and Active Labor Act (EMTALA), which passed as part of the Consolidated Omnibus Budget Reconciliation Act (COBRA) of 1985, stipulates that emergency rooms can no longer refuse to treat these patients, which results in substantial uncompensated care, bad debt, and charity expenditures that are ultimately absorbed by the insured or the taxpayer.[40–42]

It has been suggested that a more efficient deployment of resources in our healthcare system would allow preventive care to be offered universally at no or minimal incremental costs over what is already spent.[43] Needless to say, this is controversial.

HEALTHCARE REFORM AND ITS HISTORY

Before discussing the recent healthcare reform bills signed into law by President Obama, a brief review of the highlights of healthcare reform history is helpful as it puts the current state of affairs in a historical perspective. It also underlines the fact that reform is an ongoing process, and course corrections are inevitable.

In the United States, a strong dislike of "big government" prevented consideration of any significant healthcare reform until 1935.

The Social Security Act of 1935

The critical times after the Great Depression and lack of economic security required a response at the national level, which eventually came in the form of the Social Security Act, which was signed into law by President Franklin D. Roosevelt on August 14, 1935. The United States was the 35th nation to adopt such a measure to address economic security for its citizens.[44] Although the Social Security Act was not intended as a reform of the healthcare system, it did provide some assistance to the citizenry and to the states for purpose of medical care. Thirty years later, the Medicare bill was signed into law by President Lyndon Johnson on July 30, 1965, as an amendment to the Social Security Act providing health benefits to virtually all Americans above the age of 65 years. This was the first major reform of the healthcare system in the United States by way of regulatory changes. The CMS, a component of HHS, administers Medicare, Medicaid, and the State Children's Health Insurance Program (SCHIP). The Social Security Administration is responsible for determining Medicare eligibility and processing of premium payments for the Medicare program.

For years, concerns over many of the issues that were discussed in the previous sections continued to build up, and debate over the need for healthcare reform continued. In 1992 and 1993, the healthcare debate became front and center in American politics, and issues such as rising costs, access, and quality of health care were highlighted.[45–51] This culminated in an unsuccessful attempt by the Clinton administration to pass the Health Security Act of 1994. In August 1994, then Democratic Senate Majority Leader George J. Mitchell attempted to introduce an employer-friendly compromise to the earlier iterations of the bill (H.R. 3600). However, the bill failed to gain sufficient congressional support.[52]

The Clinton Reform and the Health Security Act of 1994

President Clinton envisioned a healthcare system where Americans would have choice and affordable relationships with healthcare providers. The administration recognized diminishing healthcare choices as a result of a new healthcare model known as health maintenance organizations (HMOs).[53] The goal of the legislation as defined by its proponents was "to provide for health care for every American and to control the cost of the health care system."[54] Although the Health Security Act (HSA) of 1994 focused on expansive coverage, patient choice, and retention of healthcare providers, many provisions within the act also addressed quality of care. Despite the fact that this legislation was never enacted, the ideas in the bill are still relevant today and merit some discussion.

Proposed Reform in Access to the Healthcare System

Perhaps the most significant reform that was part of HSA was expansive access to health care. HSA envisioned provisions for universal healthcare coverage to ensure that all eligible individuals had access to a health plan that delivered a comprehensive benefit package. Eligible individuals were defined as citizens, nationals, permanent residents, and long-term nonimmigrants.[55] As part of the debate over HSA, the issue of whether individuals have a right to health care was revisited at the national level.[56–61]

Proposed Reform in the Structures of the Healthcare System

The 1993 and 1994 attempts at healthcare reform contained several structural suggestions to improve healthcare quality. Legislators proposed that the National Quality Management Council develop a set of national measures of quality performance. These measures would be used to assess the provision of healthcare services and patient access. Legislators envisioned that the council would ascertain the appropriateness of healthcare services provided to consumers and measure the outcomes of these services and procedures. The council would also be responsible for gathering customer satisfaction data and examining disease prevention and health promotion. Council members would conduct periodic surveys of healthcare consumers to gather information concerning access to care and the impact of the HSA on the general population of the United States, with some emphasis placed on vulnerable populations.[54]

Such national quality measures would be thoroughly applied in order to be meaningful to agencies and legislators. Once the appropriate quality measures were identified and the information on their status within the healthcare system was acquired, the HSA policy makers envisioned that the information would be stored in computerized data banks. These data banks would provide opportunities for transparent sharing of both quality outcomes and best practices. To ensure judicious measurement and adequate implementation of other HSA provisions, policy makers recommended the establishment of the National Institute for Health Care Workforce Development. Legislators tasked the institute with development and implementation of high-performance and high-quality healthcare delivery systems.[54]

Proposed Reform in the Processes of the Healthcare System

The HSA contained many provisions geared toward measurement of quality outcomes and patient satisfaction. One such measurement process required the implementation of a national health information system. Policy makers sought to use this national health information system to gather national health information and establish quality standards. The findings would then be reported in quality report cards. The *Annual Quality Report* would contain national measures of quality for healthcare systems (hospitals, agencies, insurance providers) and would be delivered to the president and Congress annually. The Exclusion of Poor Quality Physicians Provision of the HSA allowed insurance carriers to bar poorly performing physicians from receiving reimbursement.[54]

The HSA allocated $400 million per annum to fund projects to train additional primary care physicians and physician assistants. Policy makers sought to enhance community-based generalist training for medical students, residents, and practicing physicians. Additionally, $200 million per annum would be provided for much needed training and education in managed care processes, cost-effective practice management, and continuous quality improvement.[54]

Proposed Reform in the Outcomes Measurement of the Healthcare System

Although the 1994 HSA ultimately did not pass through the 103rd Congress, there is evidence that some of the proposed quality structures and processes became reality via alternative pathways. The Agency for Healthcare Policy and Research founded by Congress in 1989 was renamed the Agency for Healthcare Research and Quality (AHRQ) in 1999. The focus and goals of AHRQ are similar to the goals of the 1994 HSA's proposed National Quality Management Council.[62] As will be discussed later in this text, many organizations today actively collect and process information on various outcomes within the U.S. healthcare system.

The Medicare Prescription Drug, Improvement, and Modernization Act of 2003

In 2003, President George W. Bush signed into law the Medicare Prescription Drug, Improvement, and Modernization Act of 2003. This was the largest single expansion of the Medicare program since its creation.[63]

The Healthcare Reform of 2010

In March 2010, President Obama signed into law the PPACA (H.R. 3590, signed on March 23, 2010). The Health Care and Education Reconciliation Act of 2010 (HCERA; H.R. 4872, signed on March 30, 2010) reconciles PPACA with the Affordable Health Care for America Act (AHCAA; H.R. 3962). This complexity was due to the U.S. Senate passing the PPACA, which was somewhat different from the AHCAA passed by the U.S. House of Representatives. To resolve the differences, the House of Representatives passed PPACA and a "fixer" bill, the HCERA, which was later passed by the Senate, in a process referred to as *reconciliation*.

The PPACA and the fixes of the HCERA, collectively referred to as the Affordable Care Act, or ACA, aim to provide affordable health care to all Americans, reduce costs, improve healthcare quality, enhance disease prevention, and strengthen the healthcare workforce.[12,64] Both acts make significant changes that directly impact the U.S. healthcare system and the quality of care provided within it.

Reform in Access to the Healthcare System

Section 1001 of the PPACA provides an amendment to the Public Health Service Act of 1944[65] and aims to improve healthcare coverage for all Americans. This amendment provides coverage for preventive health services and extends dependent coverage. It also addresses quality and cost-of-care issues within the scope of the Public Health Service Act.[12]

Section 1101 of the PPACA immediately provides access to insurance for the uninsured with preexisting conditions.[12,66] This has been a challenging aspect of healthcare coverage in the United States. Under PPACA Title II, public programs are also reformed to provide expanded coverage. A contentious part of the PPACA makes it mandatory for individuals to maintain minimum health insurance coverage. Under section 1501, it is stated that this requirement would achieve near-universal coverage. It is important, however, to emphasize that even without the individual mandate, PPACA provides expanded coverage for as many as 23 million individuals.[67]

Reform in the Structures of the Healthcare System

The PPACA and HCERA contain a multitude of structural elements to foster and encourage superior healthcare quality outcomes and mandate the creation of the Patient Centered Outcomes Research Institute. This not-for-profit institute will support comparative effectiveness research (CER), previously under the auspices of the Federal Coordinating Council for Comparative Effectiveness Research, and identify research priorities. The secretary of HHS will appoint a multistakeholder board of governors to manage the institute. The institute will use comparative healthcare economic analyses to compare and contrast the clinical effectiveness of medical interventions. However, the recommendations of the institute cannot be used to determine payment or coverage or treatment. Upon enactment, section 6302 of the PPACA will terminate the Federal Coordinating Council for Comparative Effectiveness Research, which was funded under the American Recovery Reinvestment Act of 2009.[12]

Section 10333 of the PPACA provides grants to Collaborative Care Network Programs to facilitate coordination and integration of healthcare services for low-income uninsured and underinsured populations.[12] Section 2602 of the PPACA establishes the Federal Coordinated Healthcare Office under the CMS administrator for dual eligible beneficiaries to coordinate federal and state government entities to improve quality of care and access to services for those patients who are eligible for both Medicaid and Medicare benefits.[12]

Section 3012 of the PPACA establishes the Interagency Working Group on Health Care Quality with the goal of collaboration, cooperation, and consultation between federal departments and agencies with respect to developing and disseminating strategies, goals, models, and timetables that are consistent with the national priorities. Additional responsibilities of the working group include assessing the alignment of quality efforts in the public sector with private-sector initiatives and avoiding the inefficient duplication of quality improvement efforts and resources. Many federal agencies have a seat at this table.[12]

Section 3509 of the PPACA pays special attention to women's health and establishes special offices within HHS and the CDC. The objective is to coordinate with other offices and agencies to facilitate disease prevention, health promotion, and service delivery. Similarly, section 10334 of the PPACA mandates the transfer of the Office of Minority Health to be similarly situated within the Office of the Secretary of HHS. This office will award grants and contracts to public entities to evaluate community outreach activities, language services, and workforce cultural competence in the hopes of improving healthcare outcomes in minority populations.[12]

Reform in the Processes of the Healthcare System

The PPACA calls on the secretary of HHS to create a National Strategy for Quality Improvement in Health Care. This strategy should identify national priorities and develop a strategic plan to achieve them. This national strategy and the corresponding plan is subject to periodic update.[12]

Section 3014 of the PPACA focuses on quality measurement. Under this section, the secretary of HHS may award grants and contracts to entities to support new or improve existing efforts to collect and aggregate quality and resource use measures.[12]

Section 3001 of the PPACA requires Medicare to implement value-based purchasing programs for skilled nursing facilities, home health agencies, and ambulatory surgical centers. Similarly, Medicare Advantage Plans with superior patient outcomes will also be rewarded with monetary bonuses.[12]

Section 3504 of the PPACA makes grants available for the design and implementation of Regionalized Systems for Emergency Preparedness and Response. These competitive grants are awarded by the secretary of HHS to entities to evaluate innovative models of regionalized, comprehensive, and accountable emergency trauma systems.[12]

Sections 3502 of the PPACA provide other grants including grants to establish Community Health Teams to support a Medical Home Model, awarded by the secretary of HHS, as well as grants to implement Medication Management in Treatment of Chronic Disease, awarded through the Patient Safety Research Center.[12]

Whereas some provisions seek to incentivize positive healthcare outcomes by providing rewards, there are other mandates that discourage poor-quality outcomes and wasteful practices by imposing penalties on the healthcare providers. For example, section 3025 of PPACA mandates a payment reduction for preventable readmissions and prohibits federal payments to states for Medicaid services related to conditions such as hospital-acquired infections and severe pressure ulcers resulting from poor skin care.[12]

Other mandates present within the PPACA discourage a disruption in the continuum of care, thus increasing quality patient outcomes. For example, section 1201 of the PPACA adds the Prohibition of Preexisting Conditions Exclusion by Insurance Providers section to the Public Health Services Act disallowing insurance companies to deny health insurance coverage for preexisting conditions or otherwise discriminate based on health status.[12]

These and additional elements of reform that are part of the PPACA are compared with the changes proposed in the HSA of 1994 in **Table 1-2**.

Table 1-2 Comparison of the HSA of 1994 and the PPACA with Respect to Reform in Structures and Processes[54,66]

Comparison Item	Health Security Act of 1994	Patient Protection and Affordable Care Act (PPACA)
Purpose	"..to provide health care for every American and to control the cost of the health care system."	"To make quality, affordable health care available to all Americans, reduce costs, improve health care quality, enhance disease prevention, and strengthen the health care workforce."
Proposed Reform in Structures		
Cost Effectiveness Centers		Patient Centered Outcomes Research Institute, Patient Safety Research Center
Patient Safety		Patient Safety Research Center
Collaborative Structures		Interagency Working Group on Health Care Quality, Collaborative Care Network Program
		Federal Coordinated Healthcare Office for Dual Eligibles, Medicaid Medical Home Option
Emergency/Trauma Care Programs and Centers		Trauma/Emergency Center Care and Efficiency Research Programs
Quality Improvement and Measurement Structures	National Quality Management Council	Quality Improvement Network Research Program, Value Based Purchasing Program
Women's Health Structures		Office of Women's Health
Minority Health Structures		Office of Minority Health
Payment Centers		The Center for Medicare and Medicaid Innovation—Payment Structure Evaluation
Miscellaneous Programs		Independence at Home Program
Proposed Reform in Processes		
Quality Measurement	Annual Quality Report	Gap Analysis, Grants for Developing Quality Measures, National Priorities for Quality Improvement
Reporting Quality Measures	Quality Report Card, Annual Quality Report	Quality Measure Endorsement, Public Reporting, Data Collection, Mandatory Reporting on Health Disparities
Efficiency and Delivery Incentives		Grants for Healthcare Delivery System Research, Grants for Studying Emergency Care Delivery
Preventitive Incentives		Coverage of Proven Preventative Services
Medical Home Incentives		Grants to Establish Community Health Teams—Medical Home Model
Medication Management Incentives		Grants for the Study of Medication Management

(continues)

Table 1-2 (continued)

Comparison Item	Health Security Act of 1994	Patient Protection and Affordable Care Act (PPACA)
High-Quality Rewards		Bonuses for Quality Improvement to Medicare Advantage Plans, Payment for Disease Stabilization at Mental Health Facilities
Poor-Quality Penalties	Exclusion of Poor Quality Physicians Provision	Prohibition on Exclusion for Preexisting Conditions, Nonpayment for Preventable Hospital Readmissions, Nonpayment for Hospital-Acquired Conditions (Medicaid)
Clinical Training Incentives	Primary Care and Physician Assistant Training (generalist training), National Institute for Health Care Workforce Development	Healthcare Delivery Training, Grants for Quality Improvement and Patient Safety Training
Health Disparities Processes		Exploration of Health Disparities, Mandatory Reporting on Health Disparities
Collaborative Initiatives		Bundled Payment System for Medicaid and Medicare
Legal Transparency	National Practitioner Data Bank (includes malpractice data)	Provider Screening for Fraud and Abuse, Demonstration Grants for Tort Reform, Database for False Claims, Medicare and Medicaid Compliance Programs, Demonstration Grants for Developing Alternative Medical Malpractice Processes, No Antitrust Exemption

The Supreme Court's Decision on the Affordable Care Act (ACA)

Twenty-six states challenged the constitutionality of the Affordable Care Act, and specifically the individual mandate, in the Supreme Court. On June 28, 2012, the Supreme Court largely let the ACA stand, but it did restrict the expansion of Medicaid by protecting nonparticipating states from being penalized by the Federal Government.[68]

While the decision fundamentally upholds the ACA, had it gone any other way it would not have diminished the need for a better definition of healthcare quality, better quality measurement, treating quality as an integral part of healthcare provider performance, and linking quality to cost and provider strategy. Certainly there are elements of the ACA that bring greater attention to and potential payment for quality and outcomes of care. Having those elements in place reinforces the importance of bringing greater clarity and discipline to considerations of quality in health care.

REFERENCES

1. Department of Public Health, State of Massachusetts. An Act Providing Access to Affordable, Quality, Accountable Health Care 2006.

2. National Health Expenditure Data. Centers for Medicare & Medcaid Services website. http://www.cms.gov/Research-Statistics-Data-and-Systems/Statistics-Trends-and-Reports/NationalHealthExpendData/index.html. Accessed May 17, 2012.

3. Murray CJ, Frenk J. A framework for assessing the performance of health systems. *Bull World Health Organ.* 2000;78(6):717–731.

4. OECD. Performance measurement and improvement in OECD health systems: overview of issues and challenges. In: *Measuring Up: Improving Health System Performance in OECD Countries.* Paris, France: OECD Publishing; 2002.

5. OECD. Health status: infant mortality. In: *Health at a Glance 2011: OECD Indicators.* Paris, France: OECD Publishing; 2011.

6. Anderson GF, Markovich P. Multinational comparisons of health systems data, 2008. Commonwealth Fund website. http://www.commonwealthfund.org/Publications/Chartbooks/2010/Apr/Multinational-Comparisonsof-Health-Systems-Data-2008.aspx. Published 2008. Accessed March 31, 2012.

7. OECD. Health status: life expectancy at birth. In: *Health at a Glance 2011: OECD Indicators.* Paris, France: OECD Publishing; 2011.

8. OECD. Quality of care: avoidable admissions—respiratory diseases. In: *Health at a Glance 2011: OECD Indicators.* Paris, France: OECD Publishing; 2011.

9. OECD. Health expenditure and financing: health expenditure in relation to GDP. In: *Health at a Glance 2011: OECD Indicators.* Paris, France: OECD Publishing; 2011.

10. OECD. Health expenditure and financing: health expenditure per capita. In: *Health at a Glance 2011: OECD Indicators.* Paris, France: OECD Publishing; 2011.

11. DeNavas-Walt C, Proctor BD, Smith JC, U.S. Census Bureau. Current Population Reports (P60-239): *Income, Poverty, and Health Insurance Coverage in the United States: 2010.* Washington, DC: U.S. Govenrment Printing Office; 2011.

12. The Patient Protection and Affordable Care Act. 111th Congress, 2nd Session, ed 2010.

13. NHE summary including share of GDP, CY 1960–2010; Historical National Health Expenditure Data. Centers for Medicare & Medicaid Services website. http://www.cms.gov/Research-Statistics-Data-and-Systems/Statistics-Trends-and-Reports/NationalHealthExpendData/NationalHealthAccountsHistorical.html. Accessed April 9, 2012.

14. U.S. Census Bureau. Projections of the population and components of change for the United States: 2010 to 2050. http://www.census.gov/population/www/projections/summarytables.html. Accessed March 31, 2012.

15. NHE Historical and projections, 1965–2020; Projected National Health Expenditure Data. Centers for Medicare & Medicaid Services website. http://www.cms.gov/Research-Statistics-Data-and-Systems/Statistics-Trends-and-Reports/National HealthExpendData/NationalHealthAccountsProjected.html. Accessed April 9, 2012.

16. CBO's Year-by-Year Forecast and Projections for Calendar Years 2009 to 2020; The Budget and Economic Outlook: Fiscal Years 2010 to 2020. Congressional Budget Office website. http://www.cbo.gov/publication/41880. Accessed April 9, 2012.

17. Orszag PR. CBO testimony: growth in health care costs. Delivered before the Committee on the Budget, United States Senate. Washington, DC: Congressional Budget Office; 2008.

18. Congressional Budget Office. CBO's economic projections for 2009 to 2019. http://www.cbo.gov/publication/41753. Accessed March 31, 2012.

19. Mitka M. Growth in health care spending slows, but still outpaces rate of inflation. *JAMA.* 2009;301(8):815–816.

20. Mitka M. Recession helped put brakes on growth in US health care spending for 2008. *JAMA.* 2010;303(8):715.

21. Hartman M, Martin A, Nuccio O, Catlin A. Health spending growth at a historic low in 2008. *Health Aff (Millwood).* 29(1):147–155.

22. Hartman M, Martin A, McDonnell P, Catlin A. National health spending in 2007: slower drug spending contributes to lowest rate of overall growth since 1998. *Health Aff (Millwood).* 2009;28(1):246–261.

23. Truffer CJ, Keehan S, Smith S, et al. Health spending projections through 2019: the recession's impact continues. *Health Aff (Millwood).* 29(3):522–529.

24. CMS. Factors accounting for growth in personal health care expenditures, selected calendar years 1993–2019. http://www.cms.gov/NationalHealthExpendData/downloads/PHCE_Growth_Factors.pdf. Accessed March 31, 2012.

25. Bodenheimer T. High and rising health care costs. Part 1: seeking an explanation. *Ann Intern Med.* 2005;142(10):847–854.

26. Kimbuende E, Ranji U, Lundy J, Salganicoff A, KaiserEdu.org. U.S. health care costs, 2010. http://www.kaiseredu.org/topics_im.asp?imID=1&parentID=61&id=358#9b. Published March 2010. Accessed April 10, 2010.

27. *Concentration of Health Care Spending in the U.S. Population, 2008.* Kaiser Family Foundation website. http://facts.kff.org/chart.aspx?ch=1344. Accessed March 2012.

28. CBO. *Geographic Variation in Health Care Spending.* Washington, DC: Congressional Budget Office; 2008.

29. Gottlieb DJ, Zhou W, Song Y, Andrews KG, Skinner JS, Sutherland JM. Prices don't drive regional Medicare spending variations. *Health Aff (Millwood).* 29(3):537–543.

30. Bach PB. A map to bad policy—hospital efficiency measures in the Dartmouth Atlas. *N Engl J Med.* 362(7):569–573; discussion 574.

31. Skinner J, Staiger D, Fisher ES. Looking back, moving forward. *N Engl J Med.* 362(7):569–574; discussion 574.

32. Wennberg JE, Fisher ES, Goodman DC, Skinner JS. *Tracking the Care of Patients with Severe Chronic Illness: The Dartmouth Atlas of Health Care 2008.* The Dartmouth Institute for Health Policy and Clinical Practice Center for Health Policy Research; 2008.

33. Orszag PR, Ellis P. The challenge of rising health care costs—a view from the Congressional Budget Office. *N Engl J Med.* 2007;357(18):1793–1795.

34. Fisher E, Goodman D, Skinner J, Bronner K. *Health Care Spending, Quality, and Outcomes: More Isn't Always Better.* The Dartmouth Institute for Health Policy and Clinical Practice Center for Health Policy Research; 2009.

35. Waste and inefficiency in health care. NEHI website. http://www.nehi.net/programs/17/waste_and_inefficiency_in_health_care. Accessed April 10, 2010.

36. Kelley R. *Where Can $700 Billion in Waste Be Cut Annually from the U.S. Healthcare System?* Ann Arbor, MI: Thomson Reuters; 2009.

37. Altman DE, Levitt L. The sad history of health care cost containment as told in one chart. http://content.healthaffairs.org/content/early/2002/02/23/hlthaff.w2.83.full.pdf+html. *Health Aff.* January 23, 2002. doi: 10.1377/hlthaff.w2.83.

38. Fang H, Liu H, Rizzo JA. Has the use of physician gatekeepers declined among HMOs? Evidence from the United States. *Int J Health Care Finance Econ.* 2009;9(2):183–195.

39. Orszag PR. Beyond economics 101: insights into healthcare reform from the Congressional Budget Office. *Healthc Financ Manage.* 2009;63(1):70–75.

40. Hadley J, Holahan J, Coughlin T, Miller D. *Covering the Uninsured in 2008: A Detailed Examination of Current Costsand Sources of Payment, and Incremental Costs of Expanding Coverage.* Kaiser Family Foundation; 2008.

41. Families USA. Hidden health tax: Americans pay a premium. Families USA website. http://www.familiesusa.org/resources/publications/reports/hidden-health-tax.html. 2009. Accessed March 31, 2012.

42. Families USA. Paying a premium: the added cost of care for the uninsured. http://www.familiesusa.org/resources/publications/reports/paying-a-premium.html. Revised July 13, 2005. Accessed March 31, 2012.

43. Garson A, Jr. The US healthcare system 2010: problems, principles, and potential solutions. *Circulation.* 2000;101(16):2015–2016.

44. Liu L. *Foreign Social Security Developments Prior to the Passage of the U.S. Social Security Act of 1935.* Washington, DC: Social Security Administration Historian's Office; 2001.

45. Angell M. The presidential candidates and health care reform. *N Engl J Med.* 1992;327(11):800–801.

46. Angell M. The beginning of health care reform: the Clinton plan. *N Engl J Med.* 1993;329(21):1569–1570.

47. Angell M. How much will health care reform cost? *N Engl J Med.* 1993;328(24):1778–1779.

48. Hurowitz JC. Toward a social policy for health. *N Engl J Med.* 1993;329(2):130–133.

49. Kassirer JP. The quality of care and the quality of measuring it. *N Engl J Med.* 1993;329(17):1263–1265.

50. Relman AS. Controlling costs by "managed competition"—would it work? *N Engl J Med.* 1993;328(2):133–135.

51. Relman AS. Medical practice under the clinton reforms—avoiding domination by business. *N Engl J Med.* 1993;329(21):1574–1576.

52. Rushefsky ME, Patel K. *Politics, Power & Policy Making : The Case of Health Care Reform in the 1990s.* Armonk, NY: M.E. Sharpe; 1998.

53. Clinton B. *My life.* London: Hutchinson; 2004.

54. S. 1743–103rd Congress: Consumer Choice Health Security Act of 1994. (1993). GovTrack website. http://www.govtrack.us/congress/bill.xpd?bill=s103-1743. Accessed May 2012.

55. H.R 3600–103rd Congress: Health Security Act of 1994. (1993). Library of Congress website. http://thomas.loc.gov/cgi-bin/query/z?c103:H.R.3600.IH:/. Accessed May 2012.

56. Mariner WK. Patients' rights to care under Clinton's Health Security Act: the structure of reform. *Am J Public Health.* 1994;84(8):1330–1335.

57. Olick RS. Health care reform and the right to health care. *N J Med.* 1994;91(7):472–476.

58. Morey DA. Is health care a right or a privilege? *Va Med.* 1988;115(8):380.

59. Laskin DM. Access to health care: a privilege or a right? *J Oral Maxillofac Surg.* 1987;45(4):297–298.

60. Stern SJ. Is medical care a right or a privilege? *Can Doct.* 1977;43(3):73+.

61. Stewart GT. Health care in America—privilege or right? *Lancet.* 1971;2(7737): 1305–1306.

62. AHRQ at a glance. http://www.ahrq.gov/about/ataglance.htm. AHRQ website Accessed April 10, 2010.

63. Historical background and development of social security. Social Security Administration website. http://www.ssa.gov/history/briefhistory3.html. Accessed April 10, 2010.

64. Health Care and Education Reconciliation Act of 2010. 111th Congress, 2nd Session, ed 2010.

65. Public Health Service Act, 1944. *Public Health Rep.* 1994;109(4):468.

66. Patient Protection and Affordable Care Act: preexisting condition exclusions, lifetime and annual limits, rescissions, and patient protections. Interim final rules with request for comments. *Fed Reg.* 2010;75(123):37187–37241.

67. Sheils JF, Haught R. Without the individual mandate, the affordable care act would still cover 23 million; premiums would rise less than predicted. *Health Aff (Millwood).* 2011;30(11):2177–2185.

68. National Federation of Independent Business et al. v. Sebelius, Secretary of Health and Human Services, et al. 2012; http://www.supremecourt.gov/opinions/11pdf/11 -393c3a2.pdf.

Understanding the Healthcare Organization

INTRODUCTION

The preceding chapter presented the healthcare macroenvironment, and this chapter aims to present the healthcare microenvironment of the hospital, recognizing that there are many other settings for the delivery of care. Of all such settings, inpatient and outpatient, the hospital is the largest, most complex, and most costly. For these reasons, this chapter will focus on this particular organizational context in addressing the principles of strategic planning, performance management, and organizational structure.

GOALS AND OBJECTIVES

After reading this chapter, the reader should be able to:

1. Define the organizational concepts of objectives, strategy, and structure.
2. Describe the rationale underlying the connections among objectives, strategy, and organizational structure.
3. Describe the evolution of the hospital organizational structure.
4. Understand the general similarity between the management control processes for finance and quality.

THE TYPICAL STRATEGIC PLAN FOR A HEALTHCARE ORGANIZATION

Strategic plans for healthcare organizations come in different shapes and sizes but are generally intended to reflect a sense of future direction and priorities for the organization. They often start with a statement of mission and conclude with anticipated results (performance) should the plan be implemented. Although the time horizons vary and may range from 3 years to 10 years, 5 years is a typical planning time frame. The essence of a strategic plan is the articulation of the organization's strategy; however, arriving at a feasible strategy can only result after careful attention to the organization's performance objectives and a detailed analysis of the internal and external environments. From this over-all situational assessment emerge the key strategic issues that the organization faces—often distilled from the external opportunities and threats evaluated in the context of the organization's strengths and weaknesses. It is how the organization chooses to respond to these key issues that defines the organizational strategy. This formulation of strategy is important but only sets the stage for execution (implementation) of strategy. It is in the implementation of strategy and the connection to budgets that organizations truly set themselves apart and lay the foundation for long-term viability and success.

The historic performance objectives have generally been weighted more toward financial and market measures such as profitability, revenue and volume growth, and market share. Quality, as a measure of a healthcare organization's performance, has received growing attention in recent years and in many respects is equally, if not more, central to a healthcare organization's survival. As such, it should be integrated into the overall management process and should serve to drive strategic planning in a manner parallel to that of finance.

ORGANIZATIONAL PERFORMANCE: THE TWO BOTTOM LINES

During the 1990s and early 2000s, St. Luke's Episcopal Hospital (Texas Medical Center, Houston, Texas), adopted the perspective that a healthcare organization has "two bottom lines: financial and quality." That philosophy led to the consideration of organizational performance and structure along those two equally important dimensions. The first dimension, financial, had been well developed and entrenched in the organization and in most organizations in general. The second, quality, required a great deal of attention and development to elevate it to the same level of consideration for both management and governance. It was understood that the organization would have achieved its full purpose with respect to management of performance when quality performance received the same level of priority and infrastructure support as finance.

MISSION, PERFORMANCE, STRATEGY, AND STRUCTURE

Although attending to organizational performance is critical to the long-term success of the organization, it is important to link performance to the supporting strategy and organizational structure—all in the context of the organization's mission (**Figure 2-1**).

An organization's performance objectives should ideally be derived from its mission and serve as the fundamental basis for holding healthcare organizations accountable for their stated mission. Whereas quality, or some indirect reference to quality, is in most if not all healthcare providers' mission statements, financial performance and sustainability is generally not mentioned unless indirectly captured in the notion of stewardship of the organization's assets. Thus, financial performance, although not central to a healthcare provider's "purpose," is nonetheless essential to its survival and long-term viability. In this respect, financial performance is a necessary but not sufficient condition for mission fulfillment and may be viewed as a critical means to a fundamental end: the delivery of quality health services.

Table 2-1 shows the mission statements for the *U.S. News & World Report* Honor Report Hospitals. Every year, *U.S. News & World Report* magazine ranks

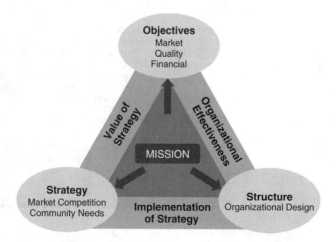

FIGURE 2-1. Connections among mission, performance objectives, strategy, and structure.

Table 2-1 Mission Statements for the Top 17 (Honor Roll) Hospitals According to the *U.S. News & World Report* Ranking in 2011

Rank	Name	Mission Statement
1	Johns Hopkins Hospital	The mission of The Johns Hopkins Hospital is to improve the health of the community and the world by setting the standard of excellence in patient care. Diverse and inclusive, The Johns Hopkins Hospital in collaboration with the faculty of The Johns Hopkins University supports medical education and research, and provides innovative patient-centered care to prevent, diagnose and treat human illness.
2	Massachusetts General Hospital	Guided by the needs of our patients and their families, we aim to deliver the very best health care in a safe, compassionate environment; to advance that care through innovative research and education; and to improve the health and well-being of the diverse communities we serve.
3	Mayo Clinic	To inspire hope and contribute to health and well-being by providing the best care to every patient through integrated clinical practice, education and research.
4	Cleveland Clinic	The mission of Cleveland Clinic is to provide better care of the sick, investigation into their problems, and further education of those who serve.
5	Ronald Reagan UCLA Medical Center	The mission of the Ronald Reagan UCLA Medical Center is to provide excellent patient care in support of the educational and scientific programs of the schools of the UCLA Center for the Health Sciences.
6	New York-Presbyterian Hospital of Columbia and Cornell	It is the mission of New York-Presbyterian Hospital to be a leader in the provision of world class patient care, teaching, research, and service to local, state, national, and international communities. The Hospital combines the best clinical and administrative practices of all its divisions, building on the strengths of each, to become the premier integrated academic health center in the United States. In concert with its two affiliated medical schools, Weill Medical College of Cornell University and Columbia University College of Physicians and Surgeons, the Hospital is committed to providing high **quality** and compassionate patient care; outstanding clinical education to physicians, biomedical scientists, and other healthcare professionals; innovative healthcare research and scientific discovery; responsible and proactive community service; unmatched service to patients, families, and visitors; and a safe work environment, competitive compensation, and the opportunity for career advancement to its staff.
7	UCSF Medical Center	Our mission—the reason we exist—is Caring, Healing, Teaching and Discovering.
8	Brigham and Women's Hospital	Brigham and Women's Hospital is dedicated to: serving the needs of our local and global community, providing the highest **quality** health care to patients and their families, expanding the boundaries of medicine through research, educating the next generation of health care professionals.

Table 2-1 (continued)

Rank	Name	Mission Statement
9	Duke University Medical Center	As a world-class academic and health care system, Duke Medicine strives to transform medicine and health locally and globally through innovative scientific research, rapid translation of breakthrough discoveries, educating future clinical and scientific leaders, advocating and practicing evidence-based medicine to improve community health, and leading efforts to eliminate health inequalities.
10	Hospital of the University of Pennsylvania	Creating the future of medicine® through: P=Patient Care and Service Excellence, E=Educational Pre-eminence, N=New Knowledge and Innovation, N=National and International Leadership.
11	Barnes-Jewish Hospital/Washington University	We take exceptional care of people: By providing world-class healthcare, By delivering care in a compassionate, respectful and responsive way, By advancing medical knowledge and continuously improving our practices, By educating current and future generations of healthcare professionals.
12	UPMC—University of Pittsburg Medical Center	UPMC's mission is to serve our community by providing outstanding patient care and to shape tomorrow's health system through clinical and technological innovation, research, and education.
13	University of Washington Medical Center	UW Medical Center improves health by providing exceptional patient- and family-centered care in an environment of education and innovation.
14	University of Michigan Hospitals and Medical Center	Excellence and Leadership in: Patient Care/Service, Research, Education.
15	Vanderbilt University Medical Center	Vanderbilt's mission is to advance health and wellness through preeminent programs in patient care, education, and research.
16	Mount Sinai Medical Center (New York)	The following Mission Statement states Mount Sinai's commitment to excellent patient care, the education of physicians and scientists, the support of innovative research, the dissemination of knowledge, the good health of the community, and the creation of a working environment conducive to individual creativity, career and personal advancement. Preamble In the context of the Jewish traditions of scholarship and charity, the Board of Trustees commits Mount Sinai to the advancement of the art and science of medicine through clinical excellence. This central mission consists of high-**quality** patient care and teaching conducted in an atmosphere of social concern and scholarly inquiry into the nature, causation, prevention and therapy of human disease.
17	Stanford Hospital and Clinics	For the benefit of our patients and the larger community, the mission of Stanford Hospital & Clinics is: To Care, To Educate, To Discover.

Note: Mission statements as they appear on the respective organization's website at the time of writing. The highlighted rows indicate that the word *quality* is explicitly mentioned in the mission statement.
Source: Data from US News and World Report. Best Hospitals 2011–12: the Honor Roll. U.S. News and World Report website. http://health.usnews.com/health-news/best-hospitals/articles/2011/07/18/best-hospitals-2011-12-the-honor-roll. Accessed on March 15, 2012.

hospitals by specialty. Hospitals that achieve excellence and top rankings in multiple specialties are included in the *U.S. News* Top Hospitals Honor Roll. What does it take to be an honor role hospital? Cutting-edge research, first-class medical training capability, and world-renowned physicians often characterize top hospitals, but how many of these hospitals' missions include the notion of quality care?

The mission statements of many honor roll hospitals emphasize research and education, and many more stress exceptional patient care, but only three hospitals, New York-Presbyterian, Brigham and Women's, and Mount Sinai, include a direct reference to "quality" care. Because an organization's mission should drive the formulation of its objectives, the notion of "quality" from the hospital's mission should be reflected in the organization's objectives.

For example, the Cleveland Clinic is ranked number four among the *U.S. News & World Report* 17 honor roll hospitals. The hospital's mission is to "provide better care of the sick, investigation into their problems, and further education of those who serve." To achieve this mission, the hospital has set the following objectives:

> To carry out this mission and foster the group practice of medicine, Cleveland Clinic must:
>
> - Excel in specialized medical care supported by comprehensive research and education.
> - Develop, apply, evaluate, and share new technology.
> - Attract the best qualified medical, scientific, and support staff.
> - Excel in service.
> - Provide efficient access to affordable medical care.
> - Ensure that Cleveland Clinic quality underlies every decision.[1]

In very general terms, the basic ingredients for organizational performance and therefore mission accountability can be reduced to answering three questions: (1) *How much* mission-related activity is done (volume)? (2) *How well* is it done (quality)? (3) *How efficiently* is it done (finance)? These three questions set the stage for determining organizational performance and mission accountability and provide the basis for setting future targets as well as initiatives designed to achieve those performance targets (**Figure 2-2**). Clearly, all three questions are connected; however, the focus of this text is the latter two: *how well* (quality) and *how efficiently* (finance).

Although *strategic plans* can take on a variety of shapes and sizes, for illustrative purposes a generic plan structure is presented in **Figure 2-3.** It is in this framework that considerations of quality performance, related strategy, and specific initiatives are integrated into the planning process with the same level of attention and

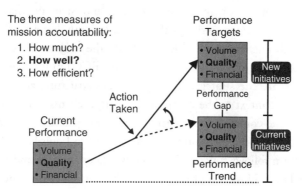

FIGURE 2-2. Organizational performance as the basis for mission accountability.

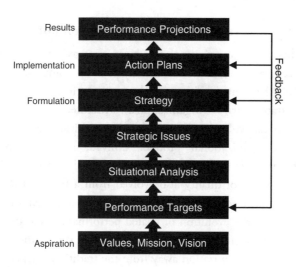

FIGURE 2-3. Generic strategic plan structure.

priority as that for financial performance—permeating the "chapters" of the strategic plan from reaffirmation of quality as essential to mission, vision, and values all the way through to the projection of quality performance that will result from the implementation of the plan. Thus, each "chapter" of the plan should explicitly address the organizational quality considerations in the context of that chapter.

Finally, the organizational structure is determined by "designing" the most appropriate "vehicle" with which to implement the selected strategy aimed at achieving the targeted performance objectives, which in turn will demonstrate mission fulfillment (Figure 2-1).

The connection of organizational strategy and structure has long been recognized in management writings that go back many decades.[2–6] In the consulting world throughout the 1970s and 1980s, the connection was recognized and promoted by the Boston Consulting Group (BCG) in its stated philosophy that objectives precede strategy, strategy precedes structure, and that all three exist within the context of the organization's purpose (mission). The origins of this concept—the connectivity of structure to strategy and objectives—may be traced back to the world of architecture, where in 1896 Louis H. Sullivan coined the phrase "form follows function,"[7] which was later adopted and promoted by his assistant Frank Lloyd Wright. Although this was challenged in a *New York Times* article in 2009[8] as an incorrect and inaccurate quotation, it is nonetheless instructive as a principle in both architecture (building design) and management (organizational design).

Structure and Strategy: Organizing to Implement

As stated earlier, the connectivity of objectives, strategy, and structure has long been recognized; however, that connectivity remains somewhat idealistic and theoretical. To the extent that in an ideal setting, performance objectives drive strategy and strategy drives (organizational) structure, it is helpful to review briefly the historical evolution of the hospital's organizational structure. As the definition of the organizational "product" evolved, from departmental operations/tasks (**Figure 2-4**) to the comprehensive medical treatment of a particular diagnosis, the concept of quality also evolved from a fragmented operational/process-related concept to a more fully defined notion of patient outcome. With that evolution came the evolution of related performance objectives, strategies, and the appropriate organizational structure. The first step in the organizational evolution moved the organization away from the traditional departmental hierarchical (tree) structure to a shared resource framework serving physician clusters oriented to specific clinical areas (**Figure 2-5**). This was the first step toward what has become the hospital service-line organization: a three-dimensional construct that better related to patients grouped by a particular diagnosis.

The history of this evolution goes back several decades. Before Diagnostic Related Groups (DRGs) (1985), the hospital was principally organized in a traditional hierarchical fashion around departments that performed specific functions—some directly related to patient care (e.g., nursing, laboratory, radiology) and some indirectly (e.g., housekeeping, dietary), and the rest were

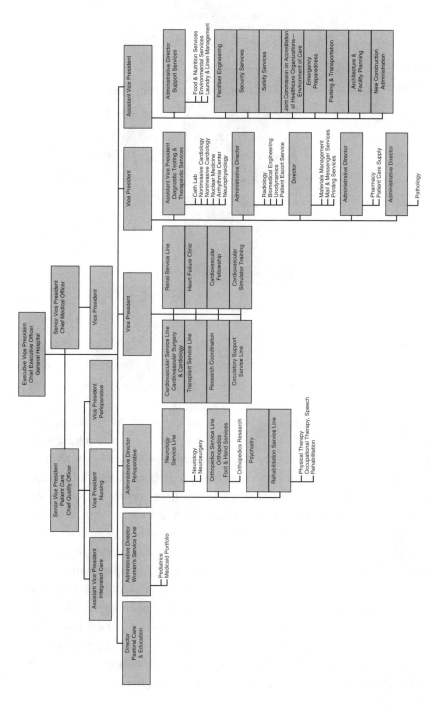

FIGURE 2-4. A traditional hospital organizational structure.

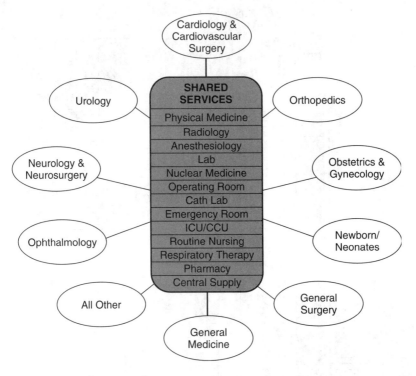

FIGURE 2-5. Physician clusters.

management overhead (e.g., finance, human resources, legal). As the prospective (DRG) payment system took hold post-1985, hospitals began to adjust their organizational structures in recognition that departments that used to be revenue centers had become cost centers in a new world of reimbursement. The concept of clinical service-line management, with service lines cutting across the old departmental structures, emerged in the late 1980s and early 1990s as a new way of thinking about the hospital organization (**Figure 2-6**). Although clearly influenced by considerations of financial performance, the concept of quality performance began to evolve from process quality within the departmental structure to outcome performance for specific classes of patients within each clinical service line (e.g., cardiovascular, orthopedic, obstetric, neurologic). Although service-line organization and management took hold, attempts at extending this to service-line management across hospitals and providers in expanding healthcare systems experienced mixed success. The two-dimensional evolution of the hospital and hospital system organization is shown in **Figure 2-7**.

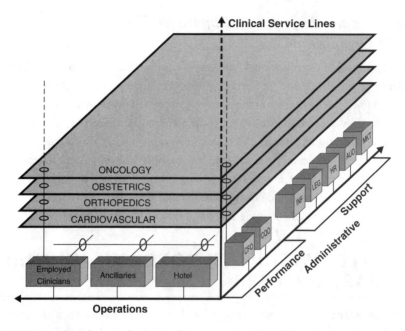

FIGURE 2-6. A hospital service-line organization. The acronyms in this figure are CFO: Chief Financial Officer; CQO: Chief Quality Officer; INF: Informatics; LEG: Legal; HR: Human Resources; AUD: Audit; and MKT: Marketing.

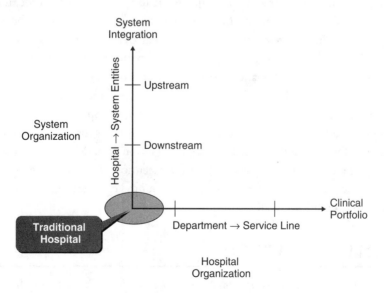

FIGURE 2-7. Hospital/system organizational evolution.

Structure and Performance Objectives: Effectiveness of the Organization

The definition of organizational "success" is captured in the stated performance objectives, and the "value" of a strategy is determined by the objectives achieved through the implementation of the strategy. However, it is the organization's ability to successfully execute the strategy that ultimately determines the "effectiveness" of the organizational structure. These connections among objectives, strategy, and structure—all motivated by the overarching mission—are reflected in Figure 2-1. Recognizing and preserving these connections will provide the necessary organizational discipline to fulfill mission and ensure long-term viability of the organization and the ongoing accountability of the leadership.

QUALITY WITHIN THE ORGANIZATIONAL INFRASTRUCTURE

Whereas financial performance and related targets have long been the principal (if not sole) drivers within the organizational strategic planning process, quality performance and targets are emerging as an equally important driver. Placement of quality performance alongside financial performance within the planning process does not require an adjustment to the framework for strategic planning but will require an adjustment to the content. Considerations of quality will then naturally flow throughout all components of the plan (Figure 2-3). In many respects, the conceptual treatment of quality performance in the plan will mirror that for financial performance: identification of the primary measures of quality performance; a historical examination of quality performance; setting of the quality performance targets; identification of the performance gaps; examination of the organization's opportunities, threats, strengths, and weaknesses associated with closing the gaps; development of initiatives for closing the gaps; and setting in motion an action plan (timetable, resource requirements, responsibilities) for execution. To a very large extent, this generic process already exists for finance, but the organizational imperative is now to extend it to quality.

CONTROL SYSTEMS

Within these overall organizational structures resided substructures that initially housed the financial reporting and control systems and more recently the quality reporting and control systems. These performance-related infrastructures contained the critical "navigational" systems designed to establish performance targets, monitor and report progress, identify variances, and guide the development of corrective action if and when the organization was "off course" with respect to its performance objectives.

A key question in this regard with respect to quality is whether the related infrastructure is adequate (particularly compared with finance) and to what extent it parallels the financial infrastructure, if appropriate.

REFERENCES

1. Mission, vision & values. Cleveland Clinic website. http://my.clevelandclinic.org/about-cleveland-clinic/overview/who-we-are/mission-vision-values.aspx. Published 2011. Accessed December 8, 2011.
2. Ansoff HI. *Corporate Strategy; An Analytic Approach to Business Policy for Growth and Expansion*. New York, NY: McGraw-Hill; 1965.
3. Buzzell RD, Gale BT. *The PIMS Principles : Linking Strategy to Performance*. New York, NY, and London: Free Press and Collier Macmillan; 1987.
4. Chaffee EE. Three models of strategy. *Acad Manage Rev.* 1985;10(1):89–98.
5. Chandler AD. *Strategy and Structure: Chapters in the History of the Industrial Enterprise*. Cambridge, MA: MIT Press; 1962.
6. Drucker PF. *The Practice of Management*. New York, NY: Harper & Row; 1954.
7. Sullivan LH. The tall office building artistically reconsidered. *Lippincott's Magazine* 57 (March 1896), reprinted in *Inland Architect and News Record* 27 (May 1896), pp. 32–34; *Western Architect* 31 (January 1922), pp. 3–11; published as "Form and Function Artistically Reconsidered," *The Craftsman* 8 (July 1905, pp. 453–458.)
8. Rawsthorn A. The demise of "form follows function." *New York Times,* May 30, 2009.

CHAPTER 3

General Concepts in Quality

INTRODUCTION

Before there was a healthcare industry, quality was recognized as a significant challenge in both the manufacturing industry and the service industry. A review of the evolution of quality from a historical perspective with an initial look at manufacturing and service industries where many of the principles of quality assurance and improvement were developed seems like the best place to start. The work performed to understand quality in the manufacturing and service industries has provided insight to many researchers and students of healthcare quality. However, there are significant differences and challenges that are unique to the healthcare industry. These call for a definition and measurement approach specific to health care and the healthcare industry.

GOALS AND OBJECTIVES

This chapter is designed to help the reader understand the history of quality and be familiar with the relevant literature and influential authors.

After reading this chapter, the reader should be able to:

1. Discuss the history of quality in the manufacturing industry.
2. Discuss the similarities of quality between the manufacturing and healthcare industries.

3. Discuss the differences of quality between the manufacturing and healthcare industries.
4. Define quality and its related domains and dimensions.
5. Discuss the role of resource utilization in the healthcare system in the quality of care.
6. Discuss some of the methodologies and tools used by healthcare organizations in quality-improvement projects.

HISTORICAL PERSPECTIVE

An understanding of the history of the quality movement in other industries, especially manufacturing, is useful in evaluating the quality movement in health care. This is particularly true where health care has "borrowed" or attempted to import quality and quality-improvement concepts from other industries.

Quality has been an important dimension in the description and assessment of products and services for comparative purposes and for judgments as to the adequacy, acceptability, effectiveness, safety, and value of products and services.

As a result of the importance of quality in manufacturing industries, most of the work on quality comes from the manufacturing literature. During the Industrial Revolution in the 18th and 19th centuries, the concept of quality underwent significant changes and became the hallmark of the manufacturing industry. Prior to this, the determination of and attention to quality was mainly achieved retrospectively through inspections of the manufactured products. This newfound attention to quality was notable for recognizing that behind every product lay a process and that to produce a quality product, it was important not only to inspect the end product (i.e., the outcome) but also to evaluate the process itself with the goal of improving it.

Before the Industrial Revolution, however, the history of quality dates back to medieval Europe where craftsmen belonged to trade unions (called *guilds*), and the guilds would approve the quality of products. These guilds had criteria for produced goods and had inspection committees that would approve a product and place a special seal of approval on the product if it met the criteria. Products were sold locally, and the reputation of the craftsman was a trademark that represented the quality of the product.[1]

Quality in this context did not have any formal definition and was based on subjective measures such as the opinion of the inspection committee members. Through apprenticeship, the craft was passed on and so was the process for making quality products.

The growth of civil societies increased the demand for certain products. The increased demand put pressure on craftsmen to increase their production capacity. At first, craftsmen hired more workers and worked alongside them in the production process. Gradually, the craftsmen went on to hire workers to keep up with the demand and transitioned themselves to a supervising role. This started the separation of front-line workers from supervisors and management. Up to this point, the interests of management were aligned with the interests of the workers. The separation of management from workers was one of the early steps that moved the responsibility of developing business strategies to management.

The factory system, a method of manufacturing developed at the beginning of the Industrial Revolution, represented the start of the quality movement during the Industrial Revolution. In this system, every individual was responsible for the development of one component of the product, whereas managers were responsible for supervising the production process. This was followed by Taylorism, a rigid factory system that was based on workflow process. Frederick Taylor, the "inventor" of scientific management, believed in work hierarchy as a means to improve the product and production processes. In Taylorism, the training of workers and product inspections were the main tools for quality assurance. Under the factory system, the entire production process occurred in one place: the factory.[1]

The importance of product quality and process quality in the United States became relevant during World War II when bullets manufactured in one state had to work in rifles manufactured in another. This coincided with the birth of new inspection techniques such as statistical process control. This technique evaluated the production process rather than the product itself and through root-cause analysis could pinpoint the deficiencies in the production process and begin to correct them. It is also worth mentioning that for the first time, products produced by two different manufacturers, or at least in two different locations, had to be compatible. The consistency of product specifications became an important hallmark of the product's quality.

The next major development in the quality movement was after World War II and started in Japan. With help from American scientists Joseph Juran and Edward Deming, Japanese managers shifted their focus from inspection of the product to the users and their needs. As a result, they succeeded in producing high-quality products and enhanced their market position by competing on product quality.[1]

American managers followed the trend, and *total quality management* came to life in the United States. This management style focused on the entire organization rather than just the product. Despite the advancements in quality practices since the Industrial Revolution, there is still no one general definition for quality. The definition of quality varies from one product to another and from one industry to the next. Even within an industry, different authorities define quality in different ways. This is in part due to the particular focus of the definition and perspective of the definers. The four perspectives recognized in the manufacturing industry include philosophical, economic, marketing, and operational.[2]

In 1947, the International Organization for Standardization (ISO) was established to facilitate international coordination of global standards.[3] The purpose of the ISO was to make products from different countries and different producers comparable. The ISO soon extended its role to making recommendations on the acceptable level of quality for different products and processes. These recommendations were derived from input by a panel of industry experts and by consumers.

Quality in Manufacturing Industries

It is fair to say that quality has a dynamic definition. This definition varies not only from industry to industry but also from time to time. In simple terms, one may think of quality as an attribute, other than price, that could differentiate two similar products. To operationalize this notion, however, is harder than it appears.

Typically, when discussing quality, one usually offers an opinion, or *judgment*, as to whether it is high, low, acceptable, and so forth. It is important, however, to recognize that this is a *two-step* process. One first needs to *measure* quality and then determine, or *judge,* whether it is high, low, acceptable, and so forth. Too often, the line between the two is lost. As will be discussed later, such evaluation of quality is the result of product/service attribute priorities determined by the individual evaluator and therefore varies from one individual to another and from time to time.

Given this history, there is no consensus on the definition of quality in manufacturing industries. This may also be a reflection of the fact that there are multiple dimensions to quality. These dimensions may well have different levels of importance and priority that can change over time. Often, the overall perception of quality may be dominated by one or a group of attributes and give the impression that the *definition* of quality has changed. If all other dimensions of quality are not significantly different among competing products, then one could argue that in fact the definition of quality in that particular context has changed. This may be a result of changes in consumer needs and expectations, changes in product functionality, or a host of other reasons. For example, early cell phones were judged by their weight, battery life, range, and so forth. Modern cell phones are judged by whether they have GPS or a high speed Internet connection. In this context, the definition of quality has changed as a result of expectations. Such changes typically manifest as a product matures and usually move from basic attributes such as functionality, reliability, and safety to efficiency and other more complex dimensions of quality.

Lack of quality standards or benchmarks make it hard to evaluate a product or compare similar products from different manufacturers. In the last 50 to 60 years, there have been attempts to establish quality standards. The ISO provides an example of such an attempt. The ISO has defined a set of standard product characteristics for a number of industries. This provides the framework for evaluating a product or comparing similar products in a given industry based on the defined standard characteristics. From the consumer's standpoint, this is very helpful given the difficulty a layperson faces in comprehending all the features of a particular product while attempting objectively to compare it with competing products. This also promotes competition and overall quality improvement in the industry. Therefore, as illustrated in the earlier example of cell phones, by use of industry standards quality can be viewed and even defined as how much the current state of a product or service is aligned with the expected state of that product or service as represented in the standards.

The process of designing and manufacturing a product is dynamic, as is the quality of the product itself. Moreover, consumer expectations for product/service quality rise as exposure to the product/service increases and the product/service matures. An acceptable level of quality when a product or service is first in its class/category to the market is relatively low compared with the acceptable quality of that same product or service after several years (see the previous cell phone example).

Another example will clarify this dynamic process. As mentioned earlier, during World War II quality gained attention as bullets made in one factory had to fit rifles made in another factory. Inspection of bullets was a way of ensuring and auditing their quality. In this context, quality meant safety and reliability, and no additional characteristics were addressed. But today, those bullets are also expected to at least travel a certain distance with some level of accuracy. At the beginning of the quality movement in the United States and at a time when Japanese products were gaining market share, American manufacturers were competing primarily on price.[3] It was soon realized that the quality of a product should be a major consideration in competitive positioning. Since then, in the manufacturing industry quality of goods has become a crucial ingredient in competition and marketing in an effort to please the consumers and protect them from annoyance.[4]

Scholarly Definitions of Quality in the Manufacturing Industries

A review of definitions of quality by scholars will provide an understanding of the complexity of this topic and will also assist in defining healthcare quality.[5]

W. Edwards Deming's definition of quality is "satisfying the customer."[5] Deming believed in customer-focused quality. Therefore, anticipating a customer's needs and expectations and "delighting"[5] customers with features and specifications are central to achieving high quality in products and services. He believed that quality is a never-ending process and should continue indefinitely.

Even though Deming's definition of quality was based on the product, he believed that managers needed to look at more than just the quality of the end product. Deming relied on statistical process control (SPC) to measure quality throughout the process of production. His goal was to create a process that had minimal variability in the final product. He classified variability into two groups: common variability and special variability. He viewed common variability as a systemic problem that could be addressed by managers, whereas special variability was due to individual differences. Deming's view of quality is a holistic one; according to his view, whole team or company should be involved in the quality process.[5] He believed that quality improvement was a dynamic and continuous process with no end. He viewed employees as a special group of customers, and therefore meeting their expectations was a quality goal as well.

Joseph M. Juran defined quality as "fitness for purpose or use."[5] The goal was to satisfy the customer, similar to Deming's goal. Fitness for purpose addresses the quality of the product or service from a design standpoint and also from the standpoint of reliability, maintainability, safety, and usability. Juran's emphasis, similar to that of Deming, was on teamwork.[5] He recognized the contribution of the human factors to quality and proposed a team approach. He defined the term *quality cost* as the cost of preventing, finding, and fixing quality problems. He also believed that quality cost could be reduced if top management was properly involved in the process. [6]

Armand Feigenbaum introduced Total Quality Control in 1951 as a framework for businesses to integrate their efforts in quality development, maintenance, and improvement.[7] In the 1970s, the work of Deming, Juran, and Feigenbaum made the foundations of total quality management (TQM). The focus of quality in TQM is on the entire process rather than just the product. This was the beginning of widespread attention to quality in all industries, including service industries. Managers began integrating quality considerations and measures into their strategic planning. TQM is a clear example of quality as a management philosophy.

Philip B. Crosby defined quality as "conformance to requirements."[5] He believed that any customer would have a set of requirements and that the manufacturer should be interested in conforming to those requirements. On the basis of this definition, he clearly viewed quality from the standpoint of the manufacturer who has to follow strict requirements to produce products that are appealing to the consumer. From the beginning, his emphasis was on "zero defects."[5] Crosby, similar to Deming and Juran, required the involvement of top management in the design and development of quality practices and products. Crosby's definition of quality is based on the known requirements of customers. Therefore, it is very difficult to use his approach in service industries, such as health care, where the requirements of customers are not completely defined.

John M. Groocock described value-based quality.[5] He defined quality as "the degree of conformance of all the relative features and characteristics of a product to all of the aspects of a customer's needs limited by the price and delivery accepted by the customer." In contrast to Juran and Crosby, Groocock saw a trade-off between quality and price.[5] He also recognized that there is more than one dimension to quality.

Each of these scholars viewed quality from a different perspective. Whereas Crosby viewed quality as a basic property of the product that can be judged by certain criteria, leaving no room for personal preferences, Juran and Deming had more respect for personal preferences of the customers. Juran, Crosby, and Deming saw quality as a marketing tool with no direct relationship between quality and price, whereas Groocock believed in a direct relationship between the two.

Dimensions of Quality in Manufacturing Industries

It has become evident that quality is rarely a unidimensional concept. More often, it is a set of attributes representing different dimensions. For example, quality of automobiles will be compared based on several different dimensions including technical, functional, and others. Whereas acceleration and fuel efficiency are the attributes of technical dimensions, user friendliness of the navigation system is a functional attribute.

Quality can have objective and subjective characteristics. Objective characteristics are measurable and can be quantified, whereas subjective characteristics are not readily measurable. Examples of objective and subjective characteristics in a product are weight and aesthetics, respectively.

David A. Garvin defines eight dimensions for quality.[4] These are

1. Performance
2. Features
3. Reliability
4. Conformance
5. Durability
6. Serviceability
7. Aesthetics
8. Perceived quality

A quality product, from one consumer's standpoint, may not have to score high in certain dimensions, whereas another consumer may demand higher scores on those dimensions. As discussed before, consumer preferences and expectations determine how a product's quality is judged. Therefore, not surprisingly, having different preferences and expectations along multiple dimensions of quality will result in the emergence of different classes of quality. These classes can be organized into levels as they represent a pyramid: the higher one goes, the stricter the expectations are.

One of the easily applicable models in industry for levels of quality is Noriaki Kano's model of quality.[8] Kano bases his model on the concept of customer satisfaction. He divides customers' needs into three categories:

1. Basic requirements: These characteristics must exist in a product or service or the customer will not stay loyal to that product or service. These requirements are the floor (minimum) for quality of a product or service.
2. Performance requirements: These requirements satisfy the consumer and have a linear relationship with the customer's satisfaction.
3. Excitement requirements: Consumers do not really expect them, but if they are there, the level of satisfaction rises. These requirements come as a surprise to the consumers.

Quality in Service Industries

This review of the history of the quality movement reveals that quality has been transformed from merely a subjective and qualitative characteristic of the end product to an expected and measurable attribute of the product and its related production process. The impact of quality considerations is felt at different levels of the production chain from top management all the way through to the consumers of the product or service.

The process of quality management has also been transformed from individual responsibilities to institutional and system responsibilities. The works of Deming, Juran, and Crosby reflect this transformation in shifting the responsibility from workers to top management and finally in creating the concept of teamwork and a sense of shared responsibility.

Despite this history, quality in service industries remains difficult to define, and methods used to measure quality in tangible products based on manufacturing processes are not always directly applicable here.

Customer expectations in manufacturing industries create specifications that will be the basis for defining a quality product. In service industries, variability of consumer expectations gives rise to the variability in services provided and so to the quality of services provided. The major relevant differences between manufacturing and service industries include[9]:

1. Services are intangible and perishable; they cannot be measured, stored, or evaluated prior to delivery.
2. Services are variable from provider to provider, customer to customer, and from time to time.
3. The service (as a "product") is for the most part inseparable from its production process (delivery) and consumption by the customer.

The best tool for measuring quality in a service industry is SERVQUAL, which uses the following dimensions for measurement[9]:

1. Tangibles, such as physical facilities including equipment and personnel
2. Reliability, delivery of service accurately and dependably
3. Responsiveness, willingness to provide prompt service
4. Assurance, delivery of a courteous, competent, and credible service with the ability to impress the customer with confidence
5. Empathy, caring for and understanding the customer

Two of these dimensions, assurance and empathy, have subcategories. The subcategories for assurance are *competence, courtesy, credibility*, and *security*. Competence relates to the professional capability to address a problem from knowledge and training standpoints. Courtesy relates to the degree of respect shown to the customer by those providing the service. Credibility relates to reputation and credentials. Security relates to feeling safe from accidents while receiving a service. The subcategories of assurance include *access, communications,* and *understanding the customer.* Access relates to the time at which the service is available. Communications relates to listening to the customer and keeping the customer informed of the expected events. Understanding the customer is reflected in the effort by a service provider to understand specific individual needs and expectations.[9,10]

Lessons from the Manufacturing and Service Industries

As the definition of quality, its assessment, and its applications vary among industries, it is important to have a framework for describing and assessing quality. This will make the definitions and characteristics of quality portable among different industries. Such a portable definition of quality across industries can be described in the form of a statement: "The quality concept is used to describe the relationship between possibilities realized and a normative frame of reference on the one hand, and to prescribe or recommend a certain form of this relationship, on the other hand."[11] This formula can be used in various contexts. For example, patients compare their expectations to what they get, and if their expectations are met they judge the care received as being of high quality. Clinicians, in contrast, will judge the care to be of high quality if the outcomes of their interventions are similar to the reported values in the medical literature.[12]

The principles of quality management in other industries can certainly be used as a guide for improvement in healthcare quality. However, because of the significant differences between health care and other industries (both manufacturing and service), no model can be directly imported from those other industries and applied to health care. The reason for the success of quality management processes in manufacturing industries is due to the nature of the manufacturing process that is directly related to the product.[13] Oftentimes, tracking of a quality deficiency could be as simple as walking back on the conveyer belt to find out where the deficiency happened. In health care, because of the complexity of the delivery system and physiologic/pathologic variations among the patients, the process and outcome are not always clearly linked.

The adoption of measurable quality practices in health care is lagging behind that of the manufacturing and service industries for several reasons worth discussing.

In comparison with manufacturing, quality is relatively new to health care. The manufacturing systems and processes had to go through several iterations of change to reach the levels of quality that we appreciate today. One of the most important reasons for this tardiness in explicitly attending to quality is the fact that for the most part, as a result of asymmetry of information, the consumer is largely unaware of what actually constitutes quality health care. This, however, changed with the publication of the Institute of Medicine (IOM) report on medical errors that shocked even the physician community.[14,15] It created an awareness that the very safety of medical care, let alone its quality, cannot be taken for granted.

Quality in modern manufacturing and service industries is not only an important attribute of the service or product but also the basis for business competition and marketing. The Profit Impact of Marketing Strategies (PIMS) project in the 1960s and 1970s[16] found that one of the most important variables to affect profitability of a business is the quality of service or product.[16] *Health care has a different payment and management structure,* and quality is not a strong basis for competition especially across geographic distances. Groocock recognized a trade-off between quality and price. The healthcare industry is primarily a third-party payer system. In this complex setting, the consumer is not the payer, and the interests of both are not completely aligned.

Health care requires greater dependence on the personal knowledge and decision-making abilities of individual healthcare providers (producers) compared with that required of the individuals in other industries. There is also a relative scarcity of standard processes for measuring the impact of a variety of strategic, operational, and financial decisions on quality. During the past 30 years, there has been an explosion of scientific and technological advancements in medical research, but translation of this science and technology to the practice of medicine has been slow.

Another reason for the delay in adoption of quality practices in health care is the fragmented healthcare delivery system, which is poorly coordinated. There are multiple levels of care, and each may involve several organizations and individuals. Different parts of this delivery system including patients, healthcare providers, payers, hospital administrators, subacute units, and pharmacies each have their own business agenda and short-term goals. There is no unifying authority among these diverse components of healthcare delivery. The process of care may involve several steps and transfers of care responsibility resulting in potential loss of information associated with the patient and the care process. The lack of standards for communication between different organizations and individuals involved in the care process may compromise overall quality. As a result of the information gaps, we often see a duplication of services and the potential for delivery of inappropriate care. *Lack of a single or properly coordinated management system for the comprehensive delivery of healthcare services is one of the major differences between medicine and other industries.*

Healthcare Industry

Health care is a service industry with a broad spectrum of services provided under the name of "health care."[17] Health care can be further divided into individual health care and public health care (**Figure 3-1**). Public health care is concerned with a vast range of topics such as epidemiology of diseases, vaccination, public policy, and insurance coverage. It also has significant consequences on individual care through policy, vaccinations, screenings, and so forth.

Individual health care similarly includes a wide range of topics ranging from medical care, to dental care, to mental health, and so forth. Under medical care, there is preventive care, medical care for acute and chronic illnesses, and sub-acute and postacute care. Each one of these categories, in turn, has subcategories. Medical care can be divided into inpatient care in a hospital setting and outpatient care in a clinic setting. Outpatient care includes doctors' offices, urgent care clinics, and day-surgery facilities. Inpatient care includes hospital admissions. Subacute and postacute care include long-term care facilities, nursing homes, and home health. The distinction of different categories makes it easier to define their scopes and implement systems to measure and improve quality of care in

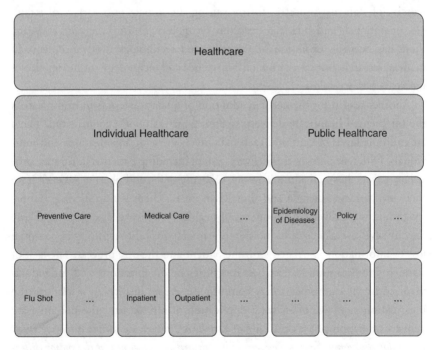

FIGURE 3-1. A depiction of the hierarchical divisions under health care.

a particular category. It is important to note that the outcomes of the entire healthcare system cannot improve as a result of efforts focused in a narrow area. Implementation of a high-quality healthcare system requires understanding these divisions and comprehensive planning and well-organized programs to cover the full spectrum of the healthcare system.

Avedis Donabedian believed that the definition of quality of health care partially depends on which part of the healthcare system is being looked at and its stakeholders.[18] But as stated by the IOM, having a shared definition for quality is critical to achieve progress and to transform the healthcare system to a high-quality industry. The discussion in this text is limited to the care provided to individuals in an inpatient hospital care setting. Although this does not cover the entire healthcare delivery system, it is the major component from a cost and resource utilization perspective and is central as a starting point for quality considerations.

Quality in the Healthcare Industry

As stated previously in this chapter, when it comes to defining and achieving quality, health care is lagging behind many other industries.

Modern quality assessment in medical care dates back to the era of Florence Nightingale. She correlated the improved outcome in the wounded to the quality of nursing care. Her use of statistical tools to interpret data is the foundation of evidence-based nursing.[19]

Ernest Codman was the first physician who formally showed interest in the modern concepts of quality of medical care and quality assessment. His concept was to follow surgical patients in hospitals and afterward evaluate the outcomes, or "end results" in his own terms, of these surgeries including any complications that arose. He hoped to establish a database that would allow him to recognize diagnostic and treatment errors and link them to the outcome. He then wanted to make these reports public to allow patients to choose where they would get care. Every other surgeon of his era was against him and his vision, and so he was fired from his staff position at Massachusetts General Hospital. He proceeded to establish his own hospital where he kept a record of all patient outcomes. He was the founder of the Hospital Standardization Program of the American College of Surgeons in 1917 (which later became the Joint Commission on Accreditation of Healthcare Organizations[20]). The basic theme in his program was reliance on competent physicians, communications among physicians, and licensing and supervision of physicians and facilities. From this perspective, it is clear that quality was seen as a product of professional judgment and not based on any specific criteria or measure.[21]

In 1952, the American College of Physicians, the American Hospital Association, the American Medical Association, and the Canadian Medical Association joined the American College of Surgeons to form the Joint Commission on Accreditation of Hospitals, which eventually was renamed in 1987 to Joint Commission on Accreditation of Healthcare Organizations (JCAHO),[21] now known as The Joint Commission, or TJC.

Perhaps the most well-known individual with major contributions to the evolution of quality and its definition in health care is Avedis Donabedian. In many respects, he was the first to recognize the systemic nature of healthcare delivery. He provided a framework for assessment of the quality of medical care by defining three elements that influence the delivery of care: structure, process, and outcome[22]:

1. Structure refers to the settings in which the care is provided.
2. Process refers to actions in giving and receiving care.
3. Outcome is the effects of care on the health status of the patient or population.[18]

Donabedian's assumptions when describing the three axes of quality are that the patient has access to health care and that the outcome for the patient depends on several transactions in the healthcare system. He believed quality of health care is a product of science and technology and their applications in health care.[23] His three elements, or dimensions, of quality—structure, process, and outcome—are only a framework for the measurement of quality in order to identify deficiencies and address them appropriately and as such provide only guidance around which many specifics must be determined.

It took several decades for government and private agencies to adopt Donabedian's framework for the measurement of quality in medical care. Interest in more precise measurement gained momentum with the advent of two critical developments:

1. The rising cost of health care and pressure from payers to objectively evaluate and compare the services offered to them and consumers.
2. The government report that identified poor quality of care as the third leading cause of death in the United States.[24]

As a result of these pressures, healthcare quality gained the public's attention and became a government priority. A new business emerged within the healthcare industry with the express purpose of defining and measuring quality of health care.

A definition for quality provides a foundation for the development of specific criteria that will determine what is expected of a high-quality healthcare system. An appropriate level of quality could be viewed as consistent achievement of desired outcomes in the healthcare system. In contrast, a poor-quality healthcare system is one that fails to increase the likelihood of desired outcomes. Based on such expectations, quality can be measured. To build a high-quality healthcare system, it is important for all involved parties, patients, clinicians, purchasers, and policy makers to adhere to a common definition for quality. In this environment, the IOM proposed the following definition for quality of health care[25,26]:

> The degree to which health services for individuals and populations increase the likelihood of desired health outcomes and are consistent with current professional knowledge.

To that end, the IOM has defined six aims (also referred to as dimensions of quality) for achieving a high-quality healthcare system. These are safety, effectiveness, patient centeredness, timeliness, efficiency, and equitability.[2] Furthermore, as will be discussed later in this text, the Agency for Healthcare Research and Quality (AHRQ) has modified Donabedian's framework to include two additional elements of access and patient experience that along with process, structure, and outcome make up five domains of healthcare quality.[27]

Healthcare managers have gone through the same stages with respect to their understanding of quality and its significance, measurement, and so forth, as their counterparts in other industries and have transitioned from quality assurance to quality improvement and then onto the current stage of quality management.[28]

Finally, it must be noted that healthcare quality can be divided into two different branches of clinical care quality and service quality. The service quality of health care includes hoteling, food service, and so forth and is an entirely different discussion from that of clinical quality, and is therefore not in the scope of this text. The focus of this text is on the clinical quality of medical care in an inpatient hospital setting.

Differences Between the Manufacturing and Healthcare Industries

It is conceivable that the understanding and knowledge gained regarding quality and quality management in the manufacturing and service industries may contribute to the progress of quality development and practice in health care. But there are important differences as one moves from concepts and practices in other industries in general to health care in particular that merit a short review.

There are at least six characteristics of the healthcare industry that distinguish it from the manufacturing and service industries. These include:

1. The asymmetry of information between provider and consumer (patient) is likely more pronounced in health care than in any other industry and therefore it makes it more difficult for the consumer to define, evaluate, and judge the quality of the service they receive.

2. The existence and influence of third-party payers and the fact that often the consumer does not pay directly for the care he or she receives make the consumer less sensitive to price and value. This obscures consideration of value received compared with other products and services where value considerations can significantly affect consumer choice. In health care, consumers seem to demand maximum quality (whether or not they know what it is) regardless of cost or value.

3. The role of the physician in health care is truly unparalleled as there is no counterpart to the physician in other industries. The physician is often not an employee of the hospital and is frequently not an owner or manager. In some respects, the physician is a "customer" of the hospital when he or she decides where to practice. Physicians are also a distribution channel (a means by which a patient is directed to a hospital). Most importantly, the physician is part of a "joint product/service" where the combination of hospital and physician makes up the complete product/service. Thus defining, evaluating, and judging quality of a complex, joint product takes on new dimensions and considerations that do not really exist in other industries.

4. In health care, the consumer (patient) is often interacting with the provider at a time of great vulnerability (unlike interaction in many other industries). That position of vulnerability, which may in part be due to asymmetry of information, anxiety, and fear, among other factors, has considerable effect on both the nature of the interactions and how quality is viewed. This interaction stresses the importance of communication between physician and patient as reflected in the patient's perception of quality as well as a potential decision by the patient to bring a malpractice suit against the provider. Effective communication is a significant mitigating factor even in the face of adverse outcomes and significantly reduces the rate of malpractice suits against physicians.[29–31]

5. Health care, for the most part, is a local/regional industry and not a global one.* Manufacturing industries, in contrast, tend to be more national and

---

*Medical tourism is currently a very small industry and is only possible for elective treatments and procedures. However, the popularity of medical tourism may be growing, which may change the healthcare industry in a small way.

global. Choice at the point of delivery of care is also limited in health care. Some healthcare interventions need to be rendered immediately, such as emergency services, although in nonurgent situations, patients may also be limited by what is available locally and by what their healthcare insurance covers.

6. Patients are as much part of the *process* of care as they are *consumers* of it. Their compliance with treatments and their perception of their medical problem as reported during history taking can actively influence the process of care. They are also the equivalent of the raw material manufacturers use to make their products. This has been recognized in health care as *case-mix,** equivalent to input variation in manufacturing. There are many biological and environmental differences among individuals so that the specifications of the input into the healthcare system vary from one case to another. The input variation in manufacturing came under control early on in the quality movement. Inescapably, patients are not built to specifications, and this difficulty is here to stay. Examples of these differences are gender, age, socioeconomic status, severity of illness, and comorbidities. Hospital organizations, by positioning themselves as tertiary and quaternary care centers, have attempted to bring case-mix (input variation) under limited control. It is not clear how successful this positioning has been.

In the manufacturing world, companies have better information about their products through their warranty and repair services, as well as parts services. While under warranty, products go back to the manufacturer, or contractors, for repairs and therefore the data is available to the organization should it be interested in improving the quality of its products. This, however, is not the case in health care. Human subjects, when born, do not come with a certificate of warranty. Even after a medical treatment or intervention—*repair* to use a manufacturing industry parallel—the work seldom comes with a warranty, with the possible exception of self-pay cosmetic procedures done in certain markets. For example, a patient may have surgery in one hospital and go to another hospital for postoperative complications. As a result, providers, hospital organizations, and medical professionals do not have data on outcomes for a significant portion of their patients.

As a result of the increase in number and impact of chronic conditions, the healthcare system has seen a growing shift from delivery of acute care to care for

---

*As healthcare providers have no control over the severity and comorbidities of their patients, risk adjustment methods are used to correct for differences in observed outcomes that are due to patient differences rather than the intervention effect.

chronic conditions. This reality in health care does not truly have an equivalent in manufacturing.* Delivery of chronic care is different in at least three respects:

1. Knowledge of prior events and interventions is crucial to decisions about the next steps. In the current system, patient records are not always available. Many times, tests and interventions are duplicated.
2. Delivery of chronic care is complex because this population is usually afflicted with more than one chronic condition, which in itself complicates the care.
3. The care of a chronic condition is more costly and complex in terms of the number of tasks and personnel involved in the care. The existence of teamwork and continuity of care is essential for delivery of proper care for chronic conditions.

Efforts to address the issue of quality in manufacturing started with quality control. Once quality control was fully developed, the next step toward higher quality was quality assurance, which included quality control. As quality assurance matured, quality improvement emerged, inclusive of quality control and assurance. Unfortunately, in health care these concepts have not fully matured. It is likely that the management teams in healthcare organizations are familiar with these terms, and most have experience with all of them. However, it does not appear that these concepts have been institutionalized into the healthcare industry. Part of this problem lies in the way quality in health care is measured. Many of the quality measures are process measures. And many of them are but a single element in the course of an encounter between a patient and the healthcare system. As such, a single process or a small group of processes cannot be expected to alter the entire outcomes of such encounters. Methods to overcome this difficulty include having well-defined encounters that include series of operations with clear beginnings and endings. The operations are broken down into processes that are linked to outcomes of the operations. These will be further discussed later in this text.

Having discussed the differences between the manufacturing and healthcare industries, it is time to review the similarities between the two.

---

*Management of legacy systems could be considered as an equivalent; however, legacy systems are a small component of the industry, and if the cost–effectiveness analyses warrant it, decisions to upgrade them can be made and implemented. Chronic conditions are a major component of the healthcare system, and these patients cannot be upgraded to newer models.

Similarities Between the Manufacturing and Healthcare Industries

As discussed earlier, David Garvin describes eight dimensions for quality in manufacturing industries. The Garvin dimensions are:[2,4]

1. Performance: Product specifications such as number or density of computer monitor or television pixels. These specifications are usually measurable characteristics that can be compared across different manufacturers.
2. Features: "Bells and whistles" associated with a product or service.
3. Reliability: "Probability of a product malfunctioning or failing within a certain time."
4. Conformance: "Product characteristics meeting established standards."
5. Durability: "A measure of product life."
6. Serviceability: "Speed, competence, and ease of repair."
7. Aesthetics: "Look, feel, sound, and other physical features of the product."
8. Perceived quality: "Lack of complete information about a product leaves the consumer to use indirect measures for comparing brands. Reputation is the primary component of perceived quality."

These eight dimensions are similar to the six IOM aims mentioned earlier. These similarities are further explored in the following paragraphs.

Performance and conformance are comparable with *effectiveness* in IOM measures. Performance can be measured and to some extent compared. There are several performance measures for every product; similarly, there are several evidence-based measures of effectiveness for many clinical services. Effectiveness of care is a somewhat loosely defined and opinion-based concept compared with performance and conformance of a manufactured product. Effectiveness can be defined as the ability and success in achieving the expected outcome. Performance is similarly focused on the outcome. An interpretation of conformance in a healthcare context would be the degree to which the processes of delivery of care for a specific condition *conform* to the established guidelines and are evidence based. In the case of a product, the resulting specifications for that end product determine *conformance*, not the nature and specifics of the manufacturing process.

Features may have some overlap with the *patient-centeredness* aim of the IOM. Features are usually additions to base product and are not essential for the product's basic functioning. In health care, examples of features can be found in additional patient amenities such as concierge service, a big-screen television in patient rooms, and massage parlors for patients; such features are not essential to achieving the desired clinical outcome. However, they may affect the perception of quality and at times are important to emphasize the patient-centeredness nature of the care being delivered; for example, a more dedicated and effective scheduling service could help patients with planning their discharges and office follow-up visits. Both in manufacturing and in health care, such features are important only to *some* consumers and usually have additional cost and will consume additional resources. In the case of the healthcare industry, the resources are finite. Allocating extra resources preferentially to the more affluent segments of the population may eventually remove resources that are accessible to the poorer segments of the population. Such resources include clinical skills or services that are limited, or treatment options that are costly.

Reliability has overlaps with *safety* and perhaps *effectiveness* among the IOM aims. Reliability is the time to failure of a product once it is being used.[2] Services, by definition, are used as they are rendered, and so reliability of a service is defined as its accuracy and dependability. In health care, two things can make a service unreliable. One is an unsafe intervention with potential adverse effects, and the other is a service that is not effective because of its lack of consistency with current standards of care. An example of an unsafe intervention is administration of medications in a hospital: if the system allows the nurses to deliver medications to the wrong patients, the medication delivery system in that hospital is unreliable. An example of an ineffective service would be in the context of a physician who does not stay current in screening his patients for colorectal cancer based on current recommendations.

Perceived quality can be viewed as *patient centeredness* in the IOM aims. Perceived quality is a reflection of how consumers view and process the "quality" of a product or service.[2] This is a subjective perception and will vary among different consumers. The patient-centeredness aim of the IOM aims reflects an attempt to involve patients and their families in decisions about their care. It relates to how competent the provider is in engaging the patients and the families and how the patients and their families perceive this involvement. Perceived quality also relates to branding of a facility or a provider. Patients and their families tend to believe that the care they receive in a reputable center or by a reputable provider is superior to the care in other places or other providers; this viewpoint is probably a reflection of experience that consumers have with a center or a provider or simply perceptions they might have. Perceived quality also relates to facilities and other services such as food services and housekeeping that are not the focus of discussion in this text.

Perceived quality from the standpoint of providers is equivalent to *efficiency*. Efficiency relates to the optimum use of resources, a characteristic that is not usually appreciated by customers because of the involvement of a third-party payer. In other words, as patients do not directly pay for the services they receive, they do not realize the value of an efficient service. An example of a patient transferred from one hospital to another will clarify this issue. The patient has had a spine MRI in the first hospital, but the MRI films are not transferred with the patient. The orthopedic surgeon in the second hospital believes that he needs to review the images quickly to decide on an operation. He will order another spine MRI to help him decide about the procedure he believes is indicated. The intended surgical procedure is performed, and the patient leaves the hospital fully functional. From the patient's standpoint, everything appears to have been performed efficiently. However, from a system standpoint, the delivered care was inefficient because of the unnecessary duplication of the MRI.

Serviceability is comparable with *timeliness* in the IOM aims. Serviceability reflects the speed with which a service or product is restored once it is broken.[2] This is equivalent to how quickly a healthcare service is rendered to an individual in need of that service.

Durability and *aesthetics* do not have an equivalent in the IOM aims. It is possible to think of the length of time a patient will be symptom free after a medical treatment as durability. However, going back to the IOM's definition, if the care provided *is consistent with current professional knowledge*, then the variability of outcome will no longer be provider dependent; rather, it will depend on the patient's biological factors and his or her compliance with medical advice, as a well as on a component of chance (luck). It is true that for certain treatments, the experience of the providers (hospital and physician) plays a significant role. For example, outcomes of prostate cancer surgery improve with the number of cases the surgeon has performed. Outcomes of treatment for leukemia are better in leukemia centers. But these outcomes are the number of complications and the success rate for the treatment and not durability. If a hip prosthesis lasts longer today than it did 10 years ago, it has to do with manufacturing of the prosthesis and not the care provided. Today, the competing prostheses will have similar life spans, and the old prostheses from 10 years ago will no longer be available in the market. How long a healthcare service for a patient lasts is the result of multiple factors. Recognition of these factors, such as treatment complications and case-mix, provides a better means of understanding quality and a more intelligent way to discuss outcomes than simply looking at the durability of the outcomes.

It is important to remember that a high-quality product might not rank on the top tier in all these dimensions.

QUALITY AND HOSPITAL CARE THROUGH THE YEARS

Over the past 200 to 300 years, hospitals have been transformed from safe houses that were meant to provide a shelter for the sick to highly technical organizations that provide care to the sickest in the population with the goal of saving lives and restoring function.[32] The shift in the role of hospitals in society along with the shift in payment systems from per diem to a prospective payment system caused a movement favoring outpatient management of the sick, creating a sicker and, consequently, more complex patient population for the inpatient setting. The intense condition of inpatient care as a result of increased average severity of illnesses among the inpatient population has also made the hospitals a place for potential errors. This increased potential for errors can cause significant harm to patients and increase the cost of medical care.

Until the mid-twentieth century, hospitals were protected from lawsuits, and hospital management was not accountable for the quality of care provided during a patient stay at its hospital. A few landmark lawsuits reversed this immunity and put more pressure on hospital managers to evaluate and measure the quality of care provided in their hospitals. The two most notable cases are *Bing v. Thunig* (1957), in which a New York court ruled that hospitals are liable for actions of their salaried employees,[33] and *Darling v. Charleston Community Memorial Hospital* (1965), where the hospital was held accountable for the negligence of its contracted physician.[34] As a result of this new legal exposure, hospitals initiated the privileging process for medical staff and licensure requirement for hospital employees.

Two major studies published in the 1990s shed light on the poor quality of hospital care and were the basis for the IOM report *To Err Is Human*.[35] These studies also provided the impetus for renewed interest and activity in the measurement and evaluation of healthcare quality.[14,15] The first study, the Harvard Medical Practice Study, was published in 1991.[34] The investigators studied the relationship between adverse events and litigation, and as part of that they reviewed data on more than 30,000 patients from 51 New York hospitals in 1984 and reported that adverse events happened in 3.7% of hospitalizations with 2.6% of errors causing permanent disability. The results of this study came as a shock to the medical community, and so another group of investigators using similar methods as those of the Harvard Medical Practice Study studied the incidence of adverse events in Utah and Colorado in 1992.[36] They reviewed the charts of 15,000 discharged patients and reported that adverse events occurred in 2.9% of the study population.

CURRENT DEFINITION OF QUALITY IN HEALTH CARE

The goal of a quality healthcare service should be to deliver more benefit than harm based on the best available information at the time of delivery of service.[36] As seen before, the IOM definition is one that is widely accepted; it defines quality of health care as: "The degree to which health services for individuals and populations increase the likelihood of desired health outcomes and are consistent with current professional knowledge."[25] This was followed by outlining the goal of achieving a high-quality healthcare system that is safe, effective, patient centered, timely, efficient, and equitabe.[26]

This definition covers the full scope of health care from public health services to the different levels of personal medical care. By using the phrase "increase the likelihood of a desired outcome," the IOM recognizes that there are known and unknown factors that affect the patient's outcome and may not be controlled by the healthcare provider. What matters is that the service should overall have a high level of benefit relative to the potential risk at the time of delivery.[36]

Whereas outcome traditionally refers to improving survival, the IOM's definition of quality highlights the importance of an individual's health expectations after care is delivered as a more comprehensive definition of outcome.[37] This implies that individuals value both longevity and functionality, although they may well have varying preferences for the mix of longevity and functionality. Thus, it is impossible to determine one single best outcome for all individuals.

Healthcare providers are responsible for delivering care that is current and evidence based, and the potential outcomes and available treatment alternatives should be clearly discussed with the patients and their families. In addition to helping patients and families decide about the treatment options, this should improve patient satisfaction with healthcare services provided and prevent unwanted and unnecessary interventions.

The IOM definition of healthcare quality also satisfies the viewpoints and interests of all stakeholders. Having a shared definition for quality is critical to the mission of quality improvement in health care. To improve the quality of health care, all stakeholders, including patients, providers, payers, and administrators, must share compatible goals and have a consistent and collaborative agenda.[26]

Dimensions of Quality in Health Care

For any quality health care provided to individuals, the general goal is to return the patient to the performance level closest to his or her condition prior to hospitalization. This, of course, should be adjusted for the physiologic losses resulting from the illness.

To that end, it must be recognized that there are several layers of providers between care provided by a physician who leads and coordinates care and care received by patients and communities. Although the clinical knowledge along with technical and interpersonal skills of healthcare providers are essential and at the core of the quality, they cannot be the only criteria for quality.[18]

Once patients access the healthcare system, practitioners' knowledge and skills are delivered to the patients through a system of care. This system consists of facilities, personnel, and processes interacting together to deliver care to patients. The patient transitions from one healthcare provider to another and from one facility to another. The actions, diagnostic tests, medications, or interventions, following the decisions of the practitioners, are the process of delivery of care. The care that the patients receive is the result of these interactions or processes. Assuming the practitioner bases his or her decisions on evidence and uses the resources appropriately, and all the system components work well, the end result should be the optimum outcome, as envisioned by the practitioner.

Quality is in the eye of the beholder, and although there might be many "beholders," the most important one is the patient. If a determinant of healthcare quality is returning the patient to his or her functional status prior to the healthcare encounter (or as close as possible), then the patient's perceptions of the quality of care he or she has received is critical.

From these discussions, it can be inferred that quality of health care is not unidimensional. The IOM recognizes that there is a gap between the current healthcare system and an optimal healthcare system and proposes six aims to transform the current healthcare system into a high-quality system. The IOM envisions a high-quality healthcare system to be safe, effective, patient centered, timely, efficient, and equitable. Each one of these aims represents a dimension and can be viewed in the context of a modified Donabedian framework of structure, process, outcome, access, and patient experience.

Health Care That Is Safe

Safety for a long time was an assumed characteristic of health care. The IOM defines patient safety as "freedom from accidental injury."[35] Even though healthcare providers were aware that errors exist, the magnitude of these errors was unknown. In 2000, the IOM reported that there are an estimated 44,000 to 98,000 deaths per year due to medical errors in hospitals.[35] This eye-opening report accelerated a number of movements in the healthcare industry to address safety problems. In addition to acknowledging the existence of major safety issues in healthcare delivery, it was generally recognized that to resolve these issues, the focus should be on the *system* of care delivery rather than on *individuals*. In other words, a broader organizational approach was needed to resolve the safety problems.

In health care, safety violations are of two major types. The first type involves the execution of an appropriate care plan that leads to an undesirable outcome, and the second type involves the selection of an inappropriate care plan, which (by definition) will not result in the desired outcome. The first type of errors are technical errors and the second type are judgment errors.[26]

The process of delivery of medical care begins with an encounter between a patient and a practitioner. The practitioner's knowledge and judgment are the foundation for safety considerations related to the prescribed diagnostic and therapeutic interventions. Major safety achievements in the past 10 years can be found in the technical arena of safety, such as medication administration or correct patient identification. Judgment errors leading to safety issues are for the most part left untouched.[38,39]

Human factors[40,*] and professional judgment are major considerations in the delivery of health care and can be the basis for many medical errors. With the exception of evidence-based[†] practice, other aspects of these considerations are still unexplored from a safety standpoint. Under evidence-based practice, it is expected that healthcare practitioners base their decisions on the available evidence.

Clearly, safety is a very important dimension of quality, but as will be discussed, it is not the only dimension. However, it is the first step in achieving a high-quality healthcare system.[26]

---

*The study of the relationships between humans, the tools they use, and the environment in which they live and work.

†Delivery of care based on available research evidence by an expert clinician with the goal of optimizing the patient's needs, values, and preferences.

Health Care That Is Effective

Effective care is the delivery of a service that is to optimize the outcome compared with that of its alternatives. Effectiveness in medical practice refers to practice of evidence-based medicine, which is the delivery of care based on available research evidence by an expert clinician while incorporating patient values in the decision-making process.[41] It is important to note that not all aspects of care have been studied sufficiently to have evidence for or against an action in every situation. That is why it is important to have an expert clinician evaluate the circumstances and draw conclusions or base actions on the best available evidence, given the patient's condition and values.

There is an overlap between the effectiveness of care and patient safety. Effective care is expected to have minimal judgment errors, leading to safe care.

Health Care That Is Patient Centered

Patient centeredness is another dimension of quality in health care. This assumes that the patient is the consumer in the healthcare system and the actions of this system should be acceptable to the patient. Attending to the expectations of patients is a goal of a quality healthcare system. Informing patients of the potential outcomes and providing them with alternatives is essential in assisting them to have realistic expectations. It is of utmost importance to communicate with the patients the uncertainties in outcomes when choosing a plan of care. Additionally, the interpersonal skills of a practitioner play a very important role in picturing the desired outcome for the patient. It is also important to realize that the resources may be limited and cost constraints may be drivers in selecting one intervention over another.

Health Care That Is Timely

The care that individuals receive should be delivered in a timely fashion otherwise there may be unwanted consequences. For example, a prolonged wait time in the emergency department may result in a patient leaving without being seen by a physician, which may result in a poor outcome. Timeliness will also improve the efficiency in the healthcare system; an example is timely transportation of patients to an MRI machine to decrease the down time on the machine.[26] It is the Donabedian *process* as well as *structure* of the delivery of care that make timeliness possible.

Health Care That Is Efficient

Efficient care is an economic measure of care and relates to the limited availability of resources associated with delivering effective care while also maximizing the benefit derived from the use of those resources. This kind of care will reduce waste in the delivery system and result in a higher value care. For example, improving safety and effectiveness of care will improve efficiency through avoiding preventable complications, resulting in fewer resources consumed.

Health Care That Is Equitable

Equity addresses the issue of access to care for populations as well as delivery of care to individuals. This partly depends on the structural context of care such as availability of hospitals and clinics, specialists, radiology, and laboratory facilities. Every individual should receive the same quality of care based on his or her needs and not based on the location of care.[26]

In nonemergent situations, for an individual to have access to these services, he or she must be able to pay for them or have coverage through a third-party payer. This brings structure and processes of the healthcare payment system into the mix.

Healthcare Outcomes

According to the Merriam-Webster Online Dictionary, *outcome* is something that follows as a result or consequence.[42] There can be many consequences to even the simplest of actions. Healthcare outcomes are defined in very much the same way. As previously discussed in the case of quality in the "Quality in Manufacturing Industries" section, outcomes, too, are seldom self-evident; they must be defined and measured. Only then can a judgment as to whether they are acceptable be rendered using some form of criteria.

Healthcare outcomes are many, and they do not have the same levels of importance. There are also different types of outcomes that can be measured along different dimensions. Two of the most important outcomes that are frequently discussed are mortality and morbidity. However, there are many other outcomes that measure important consequences of the care delivered to a patient. Examples include length of stay, cost, Medicare payment, and so forth.

One could classify mortality and morbidity outcomes under "patient's clinical status." The other outcomes that were mentioned, however, will not belong to this class. Using the six IOM aims and the fact that they represent dimensions of the care,[26] one could define outcomes that represent performance for each aim/dimension. Therefore, in addition to being dimensions of care and quality aims for a healthcare organization, the IOM aims can also represent different classes of outcomes. For example, length of stay is an outcome related to the aims of efficiency and effectiveness.

In the case of preventable mortality or morbidity, these should logically be classified as outcomes under safety, effectiveness, and perhaps equity. Addtionally, the mortality and morbidity outcomes that are not preventable should perhaps be classified under effectiveness. No care could be effective in 100% of cases, and there are mortality and morbidity that stem from physiologic differences and random events that are not foreseeable. However, the six IOM aims can be used to accommodate the majority of outcomes, including mortality and morbidity outcomes.

Finally, as was seen earlier, a single outcome such as mortality or morbidity may be associated with more than one aim. This indicates that the six dimensions are not completely independent of one another and that many outcome measures are the result of appropriate or inappropriate performance of multiple contributing factors (**Figure 3-2**).

Higher Quality and Better Outcomes

Clinical outcomes can potentially be the best measures of healthcare quality. Outcomes are the end result of care delivered to individuals and society. The

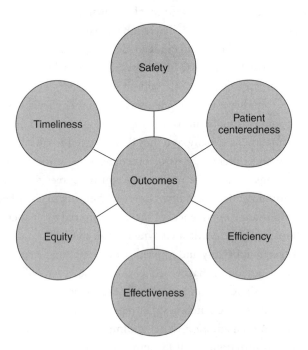

FIGURE 3-2. Outcomes can be mapped onto IOM's aims (dimensions) of quality. One outcome may be mapped onto more than one dimension.

IOM defines quality in the context of outcome. This definition links the delivery of service to the desired health outcome.[43]

Donabedian recognized that an outcome in itself is part of the quality measurement framework. There are many factors in the process of the delivery of care, some of which are not measurable. The measurable factors are processes, and the factors that cannot be measured are personal skills and judgments. Outcomes will capture both of these types of factors.[44] For example, it has been shown that centers with higher volumes of specific conditions and procedures have better outcomes for those conditions and procedures.[45] However, the exact source of the better outcomes is unknown and perhaps relates to the higher level of personnel expertise and better judgments in assessing and addressing problems related to that condition or procedure.

For a long time, healthcare providers relied on their own judgments and believed that any intervention to keep measurable clinical values in the normal range was reasonable and should be practiced; for example, the transfusion of blood products for low hemoglobin. The measure of high quality was doing anything that could be done. It is only since the introduction of outcomes research that healthcare providers are realizing that not every intervention will affect the end result (outcome).

In health care, an outcome is the end result of an intervention. The intervention would include both diagnostic and therapeutic practices as well as the process of the delivery of care. The end result could be described in terms of changes in quality of life and/or survival as well as variations in a surrogate measure such as a laboratory value or even patient perception of care.[46,47]

The desired outcome could also be described by healthcare providers through measurable physiologic values, such as survival or cholesterol level, and by measure of quality of life and functional patient-related values, such as by SF-36.* Whereas there is a considerable amount of data available on many of the physiologic outcomes, there is a scarcity of data that deal with quality-of-life outcomes. Despite improvements in the field of quality-of-life measurements, it is still in its infancy.[37] The differences between physiologic outcomes and quality-of-life outcomes are very similar to the differences between quality definition in the manufacturing and service industries. Whereas physiologic outcomes are for the most part tangible and measurable, the quality-of-life outcomes are intangible and in many respects are opinion based.

It is noteworthy that even the highest quality may not always result in desired outcomes (i.e., poor outcomes are not always the result of poor quality).[36] There

---

*SF-36 stands forMedical Outcome Study, Short Form 36 and is a reliable survey of patient health being used as a measure of quality of life.

are unknown aspects of health care other than quality of care that can affect the outcome.[44] For example, outcomes may be affected by random, uncontrollable factors as well as the capacity and ability of healthcare providers to deliver care. It may well be that the same level of care might have different results for different individuals due to factors that are not under the control of the healthcare system, such as patient factors or natural disasters.[44]

It is worth mentioning that outcome measures are also important to healthcare organizations as they can determine the current status of the organization as a tool for comparison with the organization's goals and objectives and with the organization's competitors. The baseline data can assist an organization in creating strategies aimed at improving outcomes.[13]

Shortcomings of Outcomes as Measures of Quality

In health care, similar to other industries, the ultimate goal of measuring quality is to use these measurements to improve outcomes. However, use of outcomes as a measure of quality in health care has several limitations.[22] Some of these limitations, mentioned earlier, are more fully discussed below.

Outcomes may vary not only as a result of differences in the quality of care but also as a result of *baseline* differences in individuals, such as race, sex, socioeconomic status, and payer, random chance, and disease specifics such as disease stage and case-mix.[44,48] This constitutes the input variation as discussed in the previous section "Differences Between the Manufacturing and Healthcare Industries." Case-mix adjustment methods (statistical risk adjustment) are being used to compensate for some of the differences in the patient population. As discussed before, this uncontrolled input variability in health care is in stark contrast to the ability of manufacturing industries to control inputs to their processes from suppliers and vendors.

Comprehensive measurement of outcomes is not a simple matter. Outcomes rely on large amounts of data that are not always readily available. In using existing data, care should be exercised to identify confounding factors that can potentially affect the measured outcome. Outcomes are often composite/aggregate measures and may be confounded by many known and unknown factors. If outcome data for a specific condition at a given time are collected from one hospital, it would be important to know the demographics of the patients and the makeup of providers of that hospital before using the outcome data to make comparisons with other hospitals. There are differences in the outcomes of common conditions between general hospitals and tertiary care centers due to the fact that the patients who receive care at a tertiary care center are usually sicker and have higher acuity compared with the patients at a general hospital.

Additionally, observed differences in outcomes may be attributable to an external change that happened while the impact of an intervention is being measured. For instance, better control of diabetes by primary care providers will lead to a lower rate of in-hospital mortality related to cardiac surgery.[49] If the external factor (i.e., the role of the primary care physician, or PCP, in control of diabetes) is not taken into account, it is likely that the improved cardiac surgery outcome will be incorrectly attributed to the surgeon's skills.

Outcomes data are not always available. A new intervention in its class might not have any available outcome data. In these instances, practitioners have to rely on the consensus of experts. This consensus, although valid, represents a professional judgment rather than factual data, which is the premise of outcomes. An example is the implementation of quality initiatives—such as some of TJC's core measures—with the goal of improving the quality of care. When this approach started, there was no benchmark for comparison, and policy makers had to make the leap based on professional judgments or expert opinions. The effect on the outcome for some of these interventions is debated.[50,51]

Measuring of some outcomes, such as mortality, may be relatively easy, whereas measuring of others, such as the quality of life, may be extremely difficult. Certain outcome measures may unfold over time, and it will take a long time to realize them. By the time they are available, they may not be applicable to the standards of care at the time; for example, the beneficial effects of a medication on the survival of patients with a certain condition. It will take several years to observe the patients on a medication and measure the survival benefit. Once the data are available, another new agent may be approved and used as the standard of care for treatment of that condition. The value of survival advantage of the first medication is diminished because of delay in measuring outcomes.[47]

The process of care is more sensitive than outcomes in detecting differences in quality of care and is easier to monitor and interpret.[44] The main limitation of outcomes as a measure of quality is in their application in quality improvement. Outcomes alone cannot locate the origin of the deficiency in the care delivered. Outcomes are more useful measurements of quality if they are closely linked to the other domains of access, patient experience, structure, and process in the delivery of care. Access precedes structure and process and can override a perfect performance. Through this linkage, outcome measurement can lead to actions that may improve the outcome.

Available outcome data may not be readily usable for clinical practice. For example, the highest level of clinical evidence is based on the data (outcomes) from randomized controlled clinical trials. These studies are very selective of the patients that are included in a trial. Thus, their results may not be readily applicable to the general population.[52]

Healthcare Resources, Utilization, and Quality

There exists a natural constraint on resources in a society. Such constraints, such as cost and value, introduce other concepts into the mix.[36] Without digressing into these concepts, one can still acknowledge the relationship between quality and resources; indeed without resources, there can be no quality. The healthcare industry is different from the manufacturing and service industries in that resource utilization is not necessarily controlled by supply-and-demand market forces. This is so important that it affects quality of care delivered in a healthcare system and perhaps within a healthcare organization. Therefore, it is appropriate also to think about quality and quality deficiencies in the healthcare system in terms of utilization of resources. This approach is helpful in evaluation and management of quality problems. On the basis of usage of resources, three main categories resulting in quality deficiencies are underuse, overuse, and misuse.[36]

Underuse of service is lack of access to or delivery of a service when available data support that its use will improve outcome. An example of a specific service underutilization is the underuse of stool occult blood test or colonoscopy for screening for colorectal cancer in the United States.[53] Underuse is more prevalent than expected, and access is not the only contributor to this effect. Studies of adult populations and even Medicare patients have found that up to half of the recommended services, whether for preventive care, acute conditions, or chronic conditions, are not provided.[54,55]

Overuse of service is delivery of a service when risks outweigh benefits. An example is performance of procedures for inappropriate reasons.[56] This definition has been expanded to include situations where the incremental costs of a more expensive intervention do not exceed the incremental benefits, if any.[57] Unnecessary surgery is often cited as an example of overutilization.[55] Overuse may also make the service unavailable to others who need it.

Misuse of service includes incorrect diagnoses, medical errors, and avoidable complications. Examples include hospital-acquired conditions, operations on the wrong body part,[56] and administration of a wrong medication dosage.[58] Although payers have stopped paying for such mistakes, detecting all instances of misuse in its full scope may be difficult.[57]

Quality Improvement Methodologies and Toolboxes in Health Care

Over the years, several approaches have emerged with success stories in quality improvement. Almost all originated in the manufacturing industry and were adopted, at times with some modification, by the healthcare industry. These methodologies view quality improvement as a continuous process and typically are in the form of iterative cycles.

In addition to discussing some of these methods, a brief discussion of visualization and dissemination tools for assessment of quality status is provided in the following paragraphs.

Plan–Do–Study–Act Cycle

The plan–do–study–act (PDSA) (or plan–do–check–act; PDCA) method highlights the fact that the process of quality improvement never ends and that it is a continuous endeavor of constant refinement. This cycle originates in the work of Walter A. Shewhart[59] and W. Edwards Deming[60] and has become the basis for other derivations on the original theme. A derivation of this model—find, organize, clarify, understand, and select (FOCUS) PDCA—was developed by the Hospital Corporation of America to address better the needs of a *healthcare* quality improvement project.[61] FOCUS PDCA methods were used in healthcare quality improvement initiatives such as transfusion medicine.[62]

Six Sigma

The term *Six Sigma* refers to the observation that if one can control variations such that there are six standard deviations (6σ) between the mean of a process and the nearest specification limits, there will be practically no items that fail to meet the specifications.[63] However, it is noteworthy that the variation and frequency of *defects* in the output of the healthcare system is much higher than what is dealt with in the industry.[64]

This concept of Six Sigma originated in the world of manufacturing[65] many years ago and found its way into the healthcare system. The fundamental objective is to find means of improving the quality of the output. Inspired by the PDCA/PDSA cycle, Six Sigma has a five-step methodology, referred to as DMAIC, to ensure that the desired quality is achieved[65]:

1. *Define* goals that are consistent with customer demands and enterprise.
2. *Measure* the current process for future comparison.
3. *Analyze* to verify relationship and causality of factors.

4. *Improve* the process based on the analysis of experiments.
5. *Control* to ensure that variances are corrected.

There are other related methodologies in the Six Sigma approach, such as DMADV. This methodology is typically applied to either a new process—as opposed to an established process where DMAIC is used—or where DMAIC has failed. The components of DMADV are the following[66]:

1. *Define* goals that are consistent with customer demands and enterprise strategy.
2. *Measure* and identify characteristics that are critical to quality.
3. *Analyze* to develop and design alternatives and capability to select the best design.
4. *Design*, optimize, and plan for verification.
5. *Verify*, set up pilot runs.

Lean Manufacturing

Lean manufacturing, as the term implies, is about removing waste from the production process. It was a term coined at the Massachusetts Institute of Technology inspired mainly by the success story of Toyota and the Toyota Production System (TPS).[67] The promise of cutting costs while maintaining and even improving quality has intrigued many in the healthcare industry, and hospitals seem to be the low-hanging fruits.[68] Examples of areas where "lean" principles can help improve processes in a hospital include emergency rooms,[69,70] laboratories,[71] and operating rooms.[72] Even treatment plans seem to be amenable to lean interventions, resulting in lower costs and improved quality.[73]

Visual Analysis Methods

At times, visual tools such as graphs and diagrams can be helpful in a quality improvement project. These tools add another aspect to the analytical work of addressing a quality need. A few of the more commonly used tools are discussed briefly.

A fishbone diagram is a representation of an observed effect that can be used to trace back the potential causes for that effect. It is a parallel to root cause analysis (RCA) and can be used in combination with RCA.[74]

Program evaluation and review technique (PERT), originally developed by the U.S. Navy, is an analysis tool that represents the tasks involved in completing a project.[75] It is sometimes used in combination with critical path method (CPM).

This representation style simplifies planning and facilitates decision making. It has been used in the healthcare industry as well, with some success.[76,77]

Other visualization techniques include histogram, Gantt project timeline, Pareto chart, matrix diagram, and priorities matrix.

REFERENCES

1. History of quality. ASQ website. http://www.asq.org/learn-about-quality/history-of-quality/overview/overview.html. Accessed November 5, 2011.
2. Garvin D. What does "product quality" really mean? *Sloan Management Review.* 1984; Fall:25–43.
3. Total quality. ASQ website. http://www.asq.org/learn-about-quality/history-of-quality/overview/total-quality.html. Accessed November 5, 2011.
4. Garvin DA. Competing on the eight dimensions of quality. *Harv Bus Rev.* 1987;65(6): 101–109.
5. Ghobadian A, Speller S. Gurus of quality: a framework for comparison. *Total Quality Management.* 1994;5(3):53.
6. Juran J. *Juran's Quality Control Handbook.* New York, NY: McGraw-Hill; 1988.
7. Feigenbaum AV. *Quality control: principles, practice and administration; an industrial management tool for improving product quality and design and for reducing operating costs and losses.* New York: McGraw-Hill; 1951.
8. Sauerwein EBF, Matzler K, Hinterhuber H. The Kano model: how to delight your customers. *International Working Seminar on Production Economics.* 1996:313–327.
9. Zeithaml VA, Parasuraman A, Berry LL. *Delivering Quality Service—Balancing Customer Perceptions and Expectations.* New York, NY: The Free Press; 1990.
10. Shelton P. *Measuring and Improving Patient Satisfaction.* Gaithersburg, MD: Aspen Publishers; 2000.
11. Harteloh PP. Quality systems in health care: a sociotechnical approach. *Health Policy.* 2003;64(3):391–398.
12. Harteloh P. The meaning of quality in health care: a conceptual analysis. *Health Care Anal.* 2003;11:259–267.
13. Anderson RJ, Amarasingham R, Pickens SS. The quest for quality: perspectives from the safety net. *Front Health Serv Manage.* 2007;23(4):15–28.
14. Brennan TA, Leape LL, Laird NM, et al. Incidence of adverse events and negligence in hospitalized patients. Results of the Harvard Medical Practice Study I. *N Engl J Med.* 1991;324(6):370–376.
15. Thomas EJ, Studdert DM, Burstin HR, et al. Incidence and types of adverse events and negligent care in Utah and Colorado. *Med Care.* 2000;38(3):261–271.
16. Buzzell RD, Gale BT. *The PIMS (Profit Impact of Market Strategy) Principles: Linking Strategy to Performance.* New York, NY, and London: The Free Press and Collier Macmillan Publishers; 1987.
17. Bodenheimer T. The American health care system—the movement for improved quality in health care. *N Engl J Med.* 1999;340(6):488–492.
18. Donabedian A. The quality of care. How can it be assessed? *JAMA.* 1988;260(12): 1743–1748.

19. McDonald L. Florence Nightingale and the early origins of evidence-based nursing. *Evid Based Nurs.* 2001;4(3):68–69.

20. Mallon B. E. Amory codman pioneer new england shoulder surgeon. New England Shoulder and Elbow Society website. http://www.neses.com/news.article.10.3.2009.php. Accessed November 5, 2011.

21. Luce JM, Bindman AB, Lee PR. A brief history of health care quality assessment and improvement in the United States. *West J Med.* 1994;160(3):263–268.

22. Donabedian A. Evaluating the quality of medical care. 1966. *Milbank Q.* 2005;83(4):691–729.

23. Donabedian A. *An Introduction to Quality Assurance in Health Care.* Oxford: Oxford University Press; 2002.

24. Starfield B. Is US health really the best in the world? *JAMA.* 2000;284(4):483–485.

25. Lohr KN. *Medicare: A Strategy for Quality Assurance.* Vol 1. Washington, DC: Institute of Medicine; 1990.

26. Committee on Quality of Health Care in America *Crossing the Quality Chasm: A New Health System for the 21st Century.* Washington, DC: Institute of Medicine; 2001.

27. Domain framework and inclusion criteria. AHRQ website. http://www.qualitymeasures.ahrq.gov/about/domain-definitions.aspx. Accessed November 5, 2011.

28. Luttman RJ. Next generation quality, Part 1: gateway to clinical process excellence. *Top Health Inf Manage.* 1998;19(2):12–21.

29. Johnson LJ. Sharpen communication skills to lessen lawsuit risk. *Med Econ.* 2011;88(2):48.

30. Johnson LJ. Good rapport with patients helps lessen lawsuit risk. *Med Econ.* 2011;88(1):65.

31. Virshup BB, Oppenberg AA, Coleman MM. Strategic risk management: reducing malpractice claims through more effective patient-doctor communication. *Am J Med Qual.* 1999;14(4):153–159.

32. Risse G. *Mending Bodies, Saving Souls: A History of Hospitals.* New York, NY: Oxford University Press; 1999.

33. Smith P, Shandell RE. *The Preparation and Trial of Medical Malpractice Cases.* New York, NY: Law Journal Press.

34. *Darling v. Charleston Community Memorial Hospital.* 1965. LSU website. http://biotech.law.lsu.edu/cases/medmal/darling.htm. Accessed November 5, 2011.

35. Kohn LCJ, Donaldson M. *To Err Is Human: Building a Safer Health System.* Washington, DC: National Academy Press; 2000.

36. Donaldson MS. *Measuring the Quality of Health Care.* Washington, DC: Institute of Medicine; 1999.

37. Dennison CR. The role of patient-reported outcomes in evaluating the quality of oncology care. *Am J Manag Care.* 2002;8(18 Suppl):S580–586.

38. Leape LL, Berwick DM. Five years after *To Err Is Human*: what have we learned? *JAMA.* 2005;293(19):2384–2390.

39. Altman DE, Clancy C, Blendon RJ. Improving patient safety—five years after the IOM report. *N Engl J Med.* 2004;351(20):2041–2043.

40. Weinger MB, Pantiskas C, Wiklund ME, Carstensen P. Incorporating human factors into the design of medical devices. *JAMA.* 1998;280(17):1484.

41. Sackett DL, Rosenberg WM, Gray JA, Haynes RB, Richardson WS. Evidence based medicine: what it is and what it isn't. *BMJ.* 1996;312(7023):71–72.

42. Outcome. Merriam-Webster Online Dictionary. http://www.merriam-webster.com/dictionary/outcome. Accessed April 3, 2012.

43. Chassin MR, Galvin RW, and the National Roundtable on Health Care Quality. The urgent need to improve health care quality: Institute of Medicine National Round-table on Health Care Quality. *JAMA* 1998;280(11):1000–1005.

44. Mant J. Process versus outcome indicators in the assessment of quality of health care. *Int J Qual Health Care.* 2001;13(6):475–480.

45. Halm EA, Lee C, Chassin MR. Is volume related to outcome in health care? A systematic review and methodologic critique of the literature. *Ann Intern Med.* 2002; 137(6):511–520.

46. Outcomes research: fact sheet. 2000. AHRQ website. http://www.ahrq.gov/clinic /outfact.htm. Accessed November 5, 2011.

47. Kane RL. *Understanding Health Care Outcomes Research.* 2nd ed. Sudbury, MA: Jones & Bartlett; 2005.

48. Lilford R, Mohammed MA, Spiegelhalter D, Thomson R. Use and misuse of process and outcome data in managing performance of acute medical care: avoiding institu-tional stigma. *Lancet.* 2004;363(9415):1147–1154.

49. Carson JL, Scholz PM, Chen AY, Peterson ED, Gold J, Schneider SH. Diabetes mel-litus increases short-term mortality and morbidity in patients undergoing coronary artery bypass graft surgery. *J Am Coll Cardiol.* 2002;40(3):418–423.

50. Fonarow GC, Peterson ED. Heart failure performance measures and outcomes: real or illusory gains. *JAMA.* 2009;302(7):792–794.

51. Jha AK, Joynt KE, Orav EJ, Epstein AM. The long-term effect of premier pay for per-formance on patient outcomes. *N Engl J Med.* April 26, 2012;366(17):1606–1615.

52. Fernandopulle R, Ferris T, Epstein A, et al. A research agenda for bridging the 'quality chasm.' *Health Aff (Millwood).* 2003;22(2):178–190.

53. Primary care research: studies examine ways to improve delivery of colorectal cancer screening in primary care practice. 2008; Underuse in colorectal cancer screening. AHRQ website. http://www.ahrq.gov/research/nov08/1108RA22.htm. Accessed November 5, 2011.

54. Jencks SF, Huff ED, Cuerdon T. Change in the quality of care delivered to Medicare beneficiaries, 1998–1999 to 2000–2001. *JAMA.* 2003;289(3):305–312.

55. McGlynn EA, Asch SM, Adams J, et al. The quality of health care delivered to adults in the United States. *N Engl J Med.* 2003;348(26):2635–2645.

56. McGlynn EA. Assessing the appropriateness of care—how much is too much? RAND Corporation. 1998. Rand Coporation website. http://www.rand.org/pubs/research _briefs/RB4522.html. Accessed March 2012.

57. Orszag PR. *The Overuse, Underuse, and Misuse of Health Care.* Washington, DC: Congresssional Budget Office; 2008.

58. Chassin MR. Assessing strategies for quality improvement. *Health Aff (Millwood).* 1997; 16(3):151–161.

59. Shewart WA. *Economic Control of Quality of Manufactured Product.* New York, NY: Van Nostrand; 1931.

60. Deming WE. *Out of the Crisis: Quality, Productivity and Competitive Position.* Cambridge, MA: Cambridge University Press and Massachusetts Institute of Technology; 1986.

61. McEachern JE, Neuhauser D. The continuous improvement of quality at the Hospital Corporation of America. *Health Matrix.* 1989;7(3):5–11.

62. Saxena S, Ramer L, Shulman IA. A comprehensive assessment program to improve blood-administering practices using the FOCUS-PDCA model. *Transfusion.* 2004; 44(9):1350–1356.

63. Tennant G. *Six Sigma: SPC and TQM in Manufacturing and Services.* Aldershot, England, and Burlington, VT: Gower; 2001.

64. Chassin MR. Is health care ready for Six Sigma quality? *Milbank Q.* 1998;76(4): 565–591, 510.

65. Pande PS, Neuman RP, Cavanagh RR. *The Six Sigma Way: How GE, Motorola, and Other Top Companies Are Honing Their Performance.* New York, NY: McGraw-Hill; 2000.

66. Kalra J. Medical errors and patient safety strategies to reduce and disclose medical errors and improve patient safety. Ebrary website. http://site.ebrary.com/id/10486525. Accessed April 3, 2012.

67. Womack JP, Jones DT, Roos D, Massachusetts Institute of Technology. *The Machine That Changed the World: Based on the Massachusetts Institute of Technology 5-Million Dollar 5-Year Study on the Future of the Automobile.* New York, NY: Rawson Associates; 1990.

68. Kim CS, Spahlinger DA, Kin JM, Billi JE. Lean health care: what can hospitals learn from a world-class automaker? *J Hosp Med.* 2006;1(3):191–199.

69. Ng D, Vail G, Thomas S, Schmidt N. Applying the lean principles of the Toyota Production System to reduce wait times in the emergency department. *CJEM.* 2010;12(1):50–57.

70. Dickson EW, Singh S, Cheung DS, Wyatt CC, Nugent AS. Application of lean manufacturing techniques in the emergency department. *J Emerg Med.* 2009;37(2): 177–182.

71. Bryant PM, Gulling RD. Faster, better, cheaper: lean labs are the key to future survival. *Clin Leadersh Manage Rev.* 2006;20(2):E2.

72. Cima RR, Brown MJ, Hebl JR, et al. Use of lean and six sigma methodology to improve operating room efficiency in a high-volume tertiary-care academic medical center. *J Am Coll Surg.* 2011;213(1):83–92; discussion 93–84.

73. Iannettoni MD, Lynch WR, Parekh KR, McLaughlin KA. Kaizen method for esophagectomy patients: improved quality control, outcomes, and decreased costs. *Ann Thorac Surg.* 2011;91(4):1011–1017; discussion 1017–1018.

74. Gupta P, Varkey P. Developing a tool for assessing competency in root cause analysis. *Jt Comm J Qual Patient Saf.* 2009;35(1):36–42.

75. Fazar W. Program evaluation and review technique. *American Statistician.* 1959;13(2): 646–649.

76. Lasky FD, Boser RB. Designing in quality through design control: a manufacturer's perspective. *Clin Chem.* 1997;43(5):866–872.

77. D'Aquila NW. Facilitating inservice programs through PERT/CPM. Project evaluation and review technique/critical path method. *Nurs Manage.* 1993;24(5): 92–94, 96.

Current State of Quality Measurement: External Dynamics

INTRODUCTION

Subsequent to the discussions in the previous chapters, this chapter reviews the organizations that are leaders in the field of healthcare quality. These organizations are sampled for their contributions to and leadership in the field and represent both public and private sector entities. Rather than provide consultative services or methodologies for quality improvement, these organizations have established standards for healthcare organizations. These activities range from setting regulatory mandates and accreditation procedures, to organizing meetings and forums, to offering data and funding for research.

GOALS AND OBJECTIVES

The purpose of this chapter is to provide a review of the major organizations that are involved in conducting research and defining and setting standards and measures that can contribute to the improvement of healthcare quality.

After reading this chapter, the reader should be able to:

1. Discuss the organizations involved in regulatory functions and accreditation of healthcare organizations.
2. Discuss the organizations involved in public reporting of quality performance data for healthcare organizations.
3. Discuss the organizations that provide quality performance measures.
4. Discuss the organizations that provide a forum or provide services for healthcare organizations interested in quality performance improvement.
5. Discuss the gaps in what is available with respect to the domains and dimensions of healthcare quality.

GOVERNMENT ORGANIZATIONS

The federal government is in a position to set policy for the healthcare system through legislation, to provide funding and support through grants, to offer regulatory mandates through the Centers for Medicare & Medicaid Services (CMS), and finally to offer leadership through research and public reporting of data. The key government institutions that play a prominent role in healthcare quality are described in the following sections.

U.S. Department of Health and Human Services

The U.S. Department of Health and Human Services (HHS) includes the Agency for Healthcare Research and Quality (AHRQ) and also the CMS. HHS controls public reimbursement for healthcare services (primarily Medicare and Medicaid), regulates quality performance in the healthcare system, and publicly provides performance and outcomes data. It also makes available grants for research in healthcare quality.

Agency for Healthcare Research and Quality

AHRQ provides four sets of quality measures for different healthcare providers and administrators in different settings, enabling them to measure their own quality over time and to compare themselves with national, regional, or state averages and benchmarks. The AHRQ Quality Indicators (QIs)* are composed of Inpatient Quality Indicators (IQIs), Prevention Quality Indicators (PQIs), Patient Safety Indicators (PSIs), and Pediatric Quality Indicators (PDIs).[1]

AHRQ maintains and makes available the Healthcare Cost and Utilization Project (HCUP) database, which can be used to access health statistics and information on hospital inpatient and emergency department utilization and AHRQ QIs.[2] Another tool offered by AHRQ in collaboration with other entities is the Consumer Assessment of Healthcare Providers and Systems, or CAHPS.[3] AHRQ publishes two additional useful reports: National Healthcare Quality Report (NHQR) and National Healthcare Disparities Report (NHDR). AHRQ reports, software, and other publications are available at its website.[4]

AHRQ is part of HHS and relies on the Institute of Medicine (IOM) definition of healthcare quality.

National Quality Measures Clearinghouse

The National Quality Measures Clearinghouse (NQMC), a part of AHRQ, is a database and website that lists all available evidence-based measures. In an effort to bring conformity to the selection of quality measures, its website contains detailed and clear information about quality measures. To that end, it has developed a rigorous process for evaluation of quality measures proposed by third parties (entities that submit a quality measure). If the evaluation criteria are satisfied, the measure is endorsed by NQMC.

Centers for Medicare & Medicaid Services

The Program of All-Inclusive Care for the Elderly (PACE) is a comprehensive delivery system under Medicare and Medicaid for elderly individuals in their homes. The Balanced Budget Act of 1997 (BBA [P.L. 105-33]) established PACE and mandated that the quality of care that PACE enrollees receive be monitored.[5] In 1997, CMS created a set of outcome measures and a complex system for Outcome-Based Quality Improvement (OBQI).[6,7] In addition to PACE and OBQI, CMS provides the Medicare Quality Monitoring System (MQMS) in an effort to monitor and improve the quality of care delivered to Medicare beneficiaries.[8] Some of the features of MQMS include quality indicators for the care provided to Medicare patients, utilization and outcome quality measures, characteristics of Medicare beneficiaries, and national and state-level outcomes.[9] CMS offers additional documents and resources including the CMS Quality Improvement Roadmap.[10,11]

---

*The AHRQ QIs measure quality in an outpatient or inpatient setting. All four modules rely solely on hospital inpatient administrative data.

The CMS Quality Initiative was launched nationally in 2002 with the Nursing Home Quality Initiative (NHQI) and expanded in 2003 with the Home Health Quality Initiative (HHQI) and Hospital Quality Initiative (HQI).[12,13] In 2004, the Physician Focused Quality Initiative, which included the Doctor's Office Quality Project, was developed. In 2004, the CMS Quality Initiative was expanded officially to include kidney dialysis facilities; the End Stage Renal Disease (ESRD) Quality Initiative promotes ongoing CMS strategies to improve the quality of care provided to ESRD patients. In 2005, CMS announced the launch of the Physician Voluntary Reporting Program to begin in 2006.

CMS is part of HHS. CMS also monitors patient safety and experience, health disparities, and the efficient use of health information technology. CMS uses the IOM definition of quality.

U.S. Department of Veterans Affairs

The U.S. Department of Veterans Affairs (VA) established the National Center for Patient Safety (NCPS) in 1999 to foster a culture of safety within the VA. Its goal is to achieve nationwide reduction and prevention of inadvertent care-related harm to patients through the adoption of concepts from models in fields such as aviation, nuclear power, human factors, and safety engineering.[14]

The VA is a department of the federal government and provides health care to veterans and their families. Currently, its attention to quality focuses on patient safety issues. The VA relies on The Joint Commission (TJC) for quality measures. It does not define quality explicitly and does not offer quality measures of its own.[15]

NONPROFIT ORGANIZATIONS

Healthcare quality is heavily influenced by nonprofit and independent organizations. In fact, some of the most alarming and influential reports with respect to the state of healthcare quality and outcomes have originated from this sector. Some of the more prominent nonprofit organizations are reviewed here.

The Institute of Medicine

The IOM has done its share of work in the field of quality of care, resulting in multiple publications that address issues related to quality and performance from various points of view and at different times, without specifically getting into setting of quality measures or indices. IOM's reports mainly deal with broader issues of policy and strategy.

Some of the more important reports of IOM are listed below:

- *Statement on Quality of Care*: National Roundtable on Health Care Quality—The Urgent Need to Improve Health Care Quality, January 1998.[16]
- *Measuring the Quality of Health Care*, February 1999.[17]
- *Crossing the Quality Chasm: A New Health System for the 21st Century*, March 2001.[18]
- *Envisioning the National Health Care Quality Report*, March 2001.[19]
- *Leadership by Example: Coordinating Government Roles in Improving Health Care Quality*, October 2002.[20]
- *Priority Areas for National Action: Transforming Health Care Quality*, January 2003.[21]
- *Patient Safety: Achieving a New Standard for Care*, November 2003.[22]
- *Medicare's Quality Improvement Organization Program: Maximizing Potential*, March 2006.[23]
- *Preventing Medication Errors: Quality Chasm Series*, July 2006.[24]

The IOM was chartered in 1970 as a component of the National Academy of Sciences and is a private, nonprofit organization. It provides science-based advice on matters of biomedical science, medicine, and health.[25] IOM's definition of healthcare quality is used in this text. Whereas the IOM provides a comprehensive framework for the definition of quality in health care, it does not offer specific quality measures.

National Association for Healthcare Quality

The National Association for Healthcare Quality (NAHQ) is a nongovernmental organization and publishes the *Journal for Healthcare Quality*. Instead of offering quality standards or criteria for healthcare organizations or accreditation processes, NAHQ has established a Certified Professional in Healthcare Quality (CPHQ) program, a certification process for professionals in the field of healthcare quality. NAHQ publishes practical books[26,27] and articles on current topics in healthcare quality, comments on the legislative agenda,[28] quality indicators proposed by other organizations,[29,30] and on scientific and mathematical topics relating to healthcare quality and complex healthcare systems.[31]

The Joint Commission

TJC's accreditation program (formerly the Joint Commission on Accreditation of Healthcare Organizations; JCAHO) is the most widely known quality program, perhaps because it has been delegated authority by the CMS as a requirement for reimbursement. TJC provides core measures of quality that healthcare organizations must report and has set compliance standards for those measures. The categories of these core measures are acute myocardial infarction, heart failure, pneumonia, surgical care improvement project, and pregnancy.

ORYX is the mechanism of performance measurement by and data reporting to TJC and was originally introduced in 1997.[32,33] Since then, it has become increasingly more important and has become part of maintaining accreditation by TJC.[34] TJC additionally provides the ORYX Risk Adjustment Guide. This guide treats risk adjustment as a statistical process that identifies and adjusts for variation in patient outcomes that stem from differences in patient characteristics or risk factors. In concept, this is equivalent to input variability in manufacturing. Based on the presence of risk factors at the time of healthcare encounters, patients may experience different outcomes regardless of the quality of care provided by the healthcare organization. Comparison of patient outcomes across organizations without appropriate risk adjustment can therefore be misleading. By accommodating such variations, risk adjustment facilitates a more fair and accurate interorganizational comparison.[35] ORYX data collection tools also allow collection and tracking of non-core measures that hospitals can internally report.

TJC is a nongovernmental, nonprofit organization. Its website does not offer a single, explicit, comprehensive definition for quality of health care, and the quality measures are not representative of the six IOM aims.

Institute for Healthcare Improvement

The Institute for Healthcare Improvement (IHI) focuses on identification and testing of new models of care in partnership with consumers and providers to encourage the adoption of best practices and effective innovations. IHI also aims to inspire and train the current and future healthcare workforce on quality-of-care issues. IHI has a quality improvement model based on a plan–do–study–act (PDSA) cycle.

A triple-aim approach targeting care, health, and costs by improving the experience of care, improving the health of populations, and reducing per capita costs of health care is at the core of IHI's approach.[36] Among initiatives by IHI are the 100,000 Lives Campaign and the 5 Million Lives Campaign. The 100,000 Lives Campaign aimed at saving 100,000 lives in U.S. hospitals through the adoption of six interventions.[37–39] The 5 Million Lives Campaign included six additional interventions aimed at saving lives from harm.[40]

IHI is a private, nonprofit organization and offers its services worldwide.

Hospital Quality Alliance

The Hospital Quality Alliance (HQA) is a collaborative effort between the public and the private sectors to improve the quality of care provided by the nation's hospitals through measuring and publicly reporting on that care. This collaboration includes many organizations such as CMS and the American Hospital Association and is supported by AHRQ, the National Quality Forum, TJC, and the American Medical Association, among others. It focuses on National Quality Forum–endorsed quality measures and their reporting (see the following section, "National Quality Forum").

HQA and CMS offer Hospital Compare, a website developed to report information about the quality of care delivered in the nation's hospitals.[41] These measures are limited to the treatments for heart attack, heart failure, and pneumonia, surgical care improvement, and surgical infection prevention. Whether performance improvements on these measures translate to better outcomes is unclear. One study reports that better performance in HQA measures inversely correlates with mortality,[42] but other studies find that the size of such correlations are small[43,44] and suggest that performance measures that are tightly linked to outcomes are needed.[44]

National Quality Forum

The National Quality Forum (NQF) is a private, nonprofit, public benefit corporation with the purpose of development of strategies for measurement and reporting of healthcare quality. The creation of NQF was based on a recommendation by a presidential commission in 1998 for a national forum in which health care's many stakeholders could together find ways to improve the quality and safety of the U.S. healthcare system.[45]

NQF has a process for evaluation and endorsement of voluntary consensus standards.* NQF has endorsed many quality measures proposed by different organizations and is positioning itself as a central clearinghouse for quality measures and as a national coordinator for quality discussions among different stakeholders.

Ambulatory Quality Alliance

The Ambulatory Quality Alliance (AQA) started in 2004 as a collaborative effort among the American Academy of Family Physicians (AAFP), the American College of Physicians (ACP), America's Health Insurance Plans (AHIP), and the

---

*The term *voluntary* distinguishes the standards development process from governmental or regulatory processes.

AHRQ. Its purpose is to lead an effort aimed at determining how most effectively and efficiently to improve performance measurement, data aggregation, and reporting in the ambulatory care setting.[46]

AQA collaborates with HQA and is active in data collection and reporting of quality and performance measures in different areas.[47] AQA is a nonprofit organization and does not offer a single, explicit, comprehensive definition for quality of health care.

National Committee for Quality Assurance

The National Committee for Quality Assurance (NCQA) has been active in the field of healthcare quality since 1990. Its role is to develop quality standards and performance measures for a broad range of healthcare entities and individuals, including health plans, physicians, and hospitals. A rigorous set of standards and performance criteria must be met by a health plan in order to earn NCQA's seal of approval. NCQA tracks and reports on health care delivered to individuals by the nation's top health plans.[48,49]

As one of its products, NCQA offers the Healthcare Effectiveness Data and Information Set (HEDIS™), a tool for use by health plans to measure performance on major dimensions of care and service. HEDIS consists of 75 measures in 8 domains of care. These measures are designed to provide useful information to purchasers and consumers, allowing them to compare the performance of healthcare plans.[50]

NCQA is a nonprofit organization that provides accreditation directed at health plans and certification directed at physician and hospital quality (PHQ). The PHQ certification program evaluates how well health plans measure and report the quality and cost of physicians and hospitals. NCQA also offers a definition for quality care that is narrower than that of the IOM: "Quality healthcare can be defined as the extent to which patients get the care they need in a manner that most effectively protects or restores their health. This means having timely access to care, getting treatment that medical evidence has found to be effective and getting appropriate preventive care."[51]

The American Health Quality Association

The American Health Quality Association (AHQA) is a nonprofit entity that represents quality improvement organizations (QIOs) and professionals across the country. It does not provide a definition for quality and does not offer a list of quality measures. Rather, it is a place for sharing of information regarding best practices.[52]

RAND Corporation

RAND Health offers RAND quality of care assessment tools as a comprehensive, clinically based system for assessment of quality of care. These quality indicators are based on a review of the scientific literature and on ratings by panels of experts. The RAND quality assessment tools cover 46 clinical areas and 4 functions of medicine: screening, diagnosis, treatment, and follow-up. They also cover a variety of modules related to the provision of care, such as history, physical examination, laboratory study, medication, interventions, and contacts.[53]

According to RAND, their QA tools system addresses many limitations of current quality assessment systems by relying on data from medical records rather than administrative records, establishing a scientific basis for the indicators, and targeting populations vulnerable to underutilization.[53]

The International Society for Quality in Healthcare

As the name implies, the International Society for Quality in Healthcare (ISQua) is an international organization that has members from approximately 70 different countries. Its effort is mainly focused on providing accreditation for healthcare organizations on a voluntary basis. Through a survey of standards across the three functions of leadership, support services, and service delivery, ISQua offers accreditation of an organization for the purposes of external evaluation.[54,55]

ISQua is a private, nonprofit organization that offers an accreditation program for external evaluation of healthcare organizations. It does not explicitly offer a definition of quality.

University HealthSystem Consortium

The University HealthSystem Consortium (UHC) was formed in 1984 and is a consortium of 115 academic medical centers and 257 of their affiliated hospitals comprising 90% of the nation's nonprofit academic medical centers. It creates and enhances programs and tools that assist its members in improvement of quality and safety performance. UHC programs depend on administrative databases in the academic medical centers.[56] UHC is a nonprofit, private organization.

The Leapfrog Group

The Leapfrog Group has conducted a hospital survey since 2001, which is now in its fifth version. This survey is conducted in collaboration with Thomson Reuters. The survey can be found on Leapfrog Group's website.[57] The Leapfrog Group survey includes disease-specific process and outcome measures and aims at improvement of safety, quality, and value for the employers who purchase healthcare services.[58,59] Leapfrog is a private, nonprofit organization.

FOR-PROFIT ORGANIZATIONS

Many for-profit businesses also offer their services in measurement and reporting of healthcare quality measures and outcomes. Some of the prominent organizations in this arena are reviewed here.

Det Norske Veritas

In 2008, CMS granted deeming authority to Det Norske Veritas (DNV) and essentially offered an alternative to TJC for accreditation of healthcare organizations. DNV accreditation is based on ISO 9000 standards. DNV's ISO-based accreditation, unlike TJC accreditation, does not focus on health care specifically; rather, it focuses on the quality management system.[60,61]

Although DNV is an alternative to TJC, some have suggested that use of the two together may be complementary and more productive.[60] DNV is a private, for-profit enterprise headquartered in Norway. It is active in many industries, including health care, oil and gas, shipping, food and beverages, and energy.

Thomson Reuters

After acquiring Solucient in 2008, the Thomson Corporation merged with the Reuters Group and formed Thomson Reuters. Thomson Reuters has a 100 Top Hospitals Program which uses publicly reported data and compares hospitals to similar organizations. This program offers the 100 Top Hospitals, 50 Top Cardiovascular Hospitals, and 15 Top Health Systems Awards. Winners of these awards provide the highest quality care in the most efficient manner, maintain financial stability, and have the highest patient perception of care.[62]

Thomson Reuters is a for-profit, publicly traded company and does not offer specific performance or quality measures of its own; it adopts and analyzes the widely accepted measures of TJC, AHRQ, and NQF. It issues a number of reports and publications mainly on financial and operating performance, rather than quality, and on related performance measurement.[62] In addressing quality, Thomson Reuters does not offer a broad, comprehensive definition for quality in health care.

HealthGrades

HealthGrades is a healthcare rating organization that provides ratings and profiles of hospitals, nursing homes, and physicians to consumers, corporations, health plans, and hospitals. HealthGrades compiles outcomes data from dozens of independent public and private sources and produces "report card" ratings on providers. For hospitals, the company uses information management and statistical techniques to process and risk-adjust a large volume of patient-level data. HealthGrades does not define quality explicitly, and rather than utilizing process measures it depends on mortality and morbidity data and offers "risk-adjusted" comparisons of outcomes for various hospitals.[63] HealthGrades confers an America's 50 Best Hospitals Award using this information and recognizes the better performing hospitals across the nation.

U.S. News & World Report

US News & World Report publishes an annual ranking of America's best hospitals in various specialties and also includes an honor roll for the best hospitals overall. According to an article by *U.S. News & World Report*, its ranking of hospitals seeks to inform patients who need exceptional care for rare or very complicated conditions.[64] This, according to the same article, is different from everyday care and procedures that most patients need. The *U.S. News & World Report* ranking system is based on three equally weighted parameters of reputation, mortality, and other care-related factors. Reputation is a survey of 200 randomly selected physicians for each specialty. These physicians are asked to select five centers that they believe provide the best care for "difficult cases" in their specialty regardless of cost or location. The scores are averaged for the last 3 years. *U.S. News & World Report* is a private, for-profit company.

CHANGING THE QUALITY CONVERSATION

It seems clear that significant effort is being made to address the many concerns associated with healthcare quality. Participation from government and nonprofit and for-profit organizations ensures inclusion of a variety of perspectives. Trusted and well-respected institutions such as the IOM have brought the problem into focus and have offered in-depth analyses of many of these concerns and identified pathways to address them. Funding for research in the field is available through AHRQ, and there is no shortage of quality-related measures and organizations that perform surveys and provide public reporting of those measures in the nation's hospitals.

Yet there is a clear lack of breadth and depth to the approach taken by the majority of the organizations named in this chapter. The true meaning of and sense of quality seems to be lost—often in the detail provided. One is reminded of the old adage that in many respects we seem to have "lost sight of the forest for the trees." It is natural to react to alarming reports such as the IOM study estimating the number of annual deaths due to medical errors to be as high as 98,000.[65] This is probably one of the main reasons that quality and quality measures are heavily weighted by safety concerns within the system. At the same time, identification of measures that accurately link a process to an outcome, even in safety, has proved more difficult than anticipated.

The use of administrative data is another weakness in the current system. It does not provide the details necessary to measure quality effectively and is even less effective in problem solving.[66,67]

Widely available Internet rankings of hospitals are often presented as way of identifying high-quality medical centers; however, whether these rankings reflect better outcomes is debatable.[68–71] A cursory look at the most well known of these rankings, that of *U.S. News & World Report*, reveals that reputation is the primary basis (correlation) for each center's placement on this honor list. This may be because the other two components of ranking—mortality and other care-related factors—show smaller variations among the competing hospitals when compared to repuation. Additionally, the weight of reputation on this ranking makes the overall ranking quite subjective, especially considering the fact that specialists will likely be more familiar with the centers *they* use for referring *their* difficult cases and/or with where they trained. In addition to questions about the validity of these methods, especially the reputation component, one has to wonder about the ranking's vulnerability to manipulation. Purchase of new equipment, addition of new buildings, advertising, and acceptance of referrals may translate into a higher ranking despite having little or no effect on quality as measured by outcomes. Although *U.S. News & World Report* does not claim to reflect the quality of care delivered at a medical center, it has become a quality ranking system. It is used as an advertising tool to attract patients. Hospitals on the list—especially those that made it to a prestigious position on the list—spend considerable time and resources trying to improve or at least maintain their positions.

It seems only appropriate that quality should be addressed in its full scope as defined by the IOM and not just by safety, although safety should remain a priority. Further, quality measures must be interpreted appropriately and not on face value. In the end, quality should be judged by the outcome.[72] As an example, the heart failure core measures by TJC have proved to be an expensive undertaking for U.S. hospitals and in most cases have been a success story in terms of performance improvement on those measures. However, available data suggest the outcomes have been constant among the Medicare population.[73]

REFERENCES

1. Bott J. *AHRQ Quality Indicators 101: Background and Introduction to the AHRQ QIs.* Washington, DC: AHRQ; 2010.

2. Johantgen M, Elixhauser A, Bali JK, Goldfarb M, Harris DR. Quality indicators using hospital discharge data: state and national applications. *Jt Comm J Qual Improv.* 1998; 24(2):88–105.

3. Giordano LA, Elliott MN, Goldstein E, Lehrman WG, Spencer PA. Development, implementation, and public reporting of the HCAHPS survey. *Med Care Res Rev.* 2010; 67(1):27–37.

4. Agency for Healthcare Research and Quality website. http://www.ahrq.gov/. Accessed October 26, 2011.

5. Fretwell MD, Old JS. The PACE program: home-based care for nursing home-eligible individuals. *N C Med J.* 2011;72(3):209–211.

6. Branham CN. Frequently asked questions about OBQM/OBQI. *Home Healthc Nurse.* 2002;20(8):488–490.

7. Rosati RJ. The history of quality measurement in home health care. *Clin Geriatr Med.* 2009;25(1):121–134, vii–viii.

8. Kuo S, Fleming BB, Gittings NS, et al. Trends in care practices and outcomes among Medicare beneficiaries with diabetes. *Am J Prev Med.* 2005;29(5):396–403.

9. Centers for Medicare & Medicaid Services. *The Medicare Quality Monitoring System (MQMS).* 2006.

10. CMS unveils "Quality Improvement Roadmap." *Hosp Outlook.* 2005;8(3):8–9.

11. Straube B. The CMS Quality Roadmap: quality plus efficiency. *Health Aff (Millwood).* 2005;Suppl Web Exclusives:W5-555–557.

12. Harris Y, Clauser SB. Achieving improvement through nursing home quality measurement. *Health Care Financ Rev.* 2002;23(4):5–18.

13. Elliott B. Pay for performance and the hospital quality initiative. *Del Med J.* 2005; 77(8):289–296.

14. Heget JR, Bagian JP, Lee CZ, Gosbee JW. John M. Eisenberg Patient Safety Awards. System innovation: Veterans Health Administration National Center for Patient Safety. *Jt Comm J Qual Improv.* 2002;28(12):660–665.

15. McQueen L, Mittman BS, Demakis JG. Overview of the Veterans Health Administration (VHA) Quality Enhancement Research Initiative (QUERI). *J Am Med Inform Assoc.* 2004;11(5):339–343.

16. National Roundtable on Health Care Quality. *Statement on Quality of Care.* Washington, DC: Institute of Medicine; 1998.

17. Donaldson MS. *Measuring the Quality of Health Care.* Washington, DC: Institute of Medicine; 1999.

18. Committee on Quality of Health Care in America. *Crossing the Quality Chasm: A New Health System for the 21st Century.* Washington, DC: Institute of Medicine; 2001.

19. Hurtado MP, Swift EK, Corrigan JM. *Envisioning the National Health Care Quality Report.* Washington, DC: Institute of Medicine; 2001.

20. Corrigan JM, Eden J, Smith BM. *Leadership by Example: Coordinating Government Roles in Improving Health Care Quality.* Washington, DC: Institute of Medicine; 2002.

21. Adams K, Corrigan JM. *Priority Areas for National Action: Transforming Health Care Quality.* Washington, DC: Institute of Medicine; 2003.

22. Aspden P, Corrigan JM, Wolcott J, Erickson SM. *Patient Safety: Achieving a New Standard for Care.* Washington, DC: Institute of Medicine; 2003.

23. Committee on Redesigning Health Insurance Performance Measures, Performance Improvement. *Medicare's Quality Improvement Organization Program: Maximizing Potential.* Washington, DC: Institute of Medicine; 2006.

24. Committee on Preventing Medication Errors, Aspden P, Wolcott J, Bootman JL, Cronenwett LR. *Preventing Medication Errors: Quality Chasm Series.* Washington, DC: Institute of Medicine; 2006.

25. About the IOM. Institute of Medicine website. http://www.iom.edu/CMS/About -IOM.aspx. Accessed May 4, 2009.

26. Dlugacz YD, Restifo A, Greenwood A. *The Quality Handbook for Health Care Organizations: A Manager's Guide to Tools and Programs.* San Francisco, CA: Jossey-Bass; 2004.

27. Graban M. *Lean Hospitals: Improving Quality, Patient Safety, and Employee Satisfaction.* Boca Raton, FL: CRC Press; 2009.

28. Vemula R, Robyn AR, Al-Assaf AF. Making the Patient Safety and Quality Improvement Act of 2005 work. *J Healthc Qual.* 2007;29(4):6–10.

29. de Koning H, Verver JP, van den HJ, Bisgaard S, Does RJ. Lean six sigma in healthcare. *J Healthc Qual.* 2006;28(2):4–11.

30. Hart J, Sweeney G. Integrating patient safety indicators into patient safety programs. *J Healthc Qual.* 2006;28(6):18–28.

31. Benson H. Chaos and complexity: applications for healthcare quality and patient safety. *J Healthc Qual.* 2005;27(5):4–10.

32. Lee KY, McGreevey C. Using comparison charts to assess performance measurement data. *Jt Comm J Qual Improv.* 2002;28(3):129–138.

33. Muri JH. The Joint Commission's ORYX initiative: implications for perinatal nursing and care. *J Perinat Neonatal Nurs.* 1998;12(1):1–10; quiz 81-13.

34. TJC readies new standard for ORYX measures. *Hosp Peer Rev.* 2011;36(9): 106–108.

35. ORYX risk adjustment guide. Joint Commission website. http://www.jointcommission .org/assets/1/18/RA_Guide_Risk_Model.pdf. Accessed October 26, 2011.

36. Berwick DM, Nolan TW, Whittington J. The triple aim: care, health, and cost. *Health Aff (Millwood).* 2008;27(3):759–769.

37. Berwick DM, Hackbarth AD, McCannon CJ. IHI replies to "The 100,000 Lives Campaign: a scientific and policy review." *Jt Comm J Qual Patient Saf.* 2006;32(11): 628–630; discussion 631-623.

38. Berwick DM, Calkins DR, McCannon CJ, Hackbarth AD. The 100,000 lives campaign: setting a goal and a deadline for improving health care quality. *JAMA.* 2006;295(3):324–327.

39. IHI proposes six patient safety goals to prevent 100,000 annual deaths. *Qual Lett Healthc Lead.* 2005;17(1):11–12.

40. Gold JA. The 5 Million Lives Campaign: preventing medical harm in Wisconsin and the nation. *WMJ.* 2008;107(5):270–271.

41. Hospital Compare – a quality tool provided by Medicare. HHS website. http://www .hospitalcompare.hhs.gov. Accessed October 26, 2011.

42. Jha AK, Orav EJ, Li Z, Epstein AM. The inverse relationship between mortality rates and performance in the Hospital Quality Alliance measures. *Health Aff (Millwood).* 2007;26(4):1104–1110.

43. Jha AK, Li Z, Orav EJ, Epstein AM. Care in U.S. hospitals—the Hospital Quality Alliance program. *N Engl J Med.* 2005;353(3):265–274.

44. Werner RM, Bradlow ET. Relationship between Medicare's hospital compare performance measures and mortality rates. *JAMA.* 2006;296(22):2694–2702.

45. Miller T, Leatherman S. The National Quality Forum: a 'me-too' or a breakthrough in quality measurement and reporting? *Health Aff (Millwood).* 1999;18(6):233–237.

46. AQA releases ambulatory quality measures. *Med Health.* 2005;59(16):3–4.

47. AQA, HQA collaborate on national quality strategy. *Healthcare Benchmarks Qual Improv.* 2006;13(10):115–117.

48. Bell D, Brandt EN, Jr. Accreditation by the National Committee on Quality Assurance (NCQA): a description. *J Okla State Med Assoc.* 1999;92(5):234–237.

49. Morrissey J. NCQA (National Committee for Quality Assurance) pilot project aims to make measures comparable, accurate. *Mod Healthc.* 1995;25(12):60, 62.

50. NCQA. What is HEDIS? NCQA website. http://www.ncqa.org/tabid/187/Default .aspx. Accessed November 26, 2011.

51. NCQA. Report cards. NCQA website. http://www.ncqa.org/tabid/60/Default.aspx. Accessed October 26, 2011.

52. Schulke DG, Krantzberg E, Grant J. Introduction: Medicare quality improvement organizations—activities and partnerships. *J Manag Care Pharm.* 2007;13(6 Suppl B): S3–6.

53. Kerr EA, Health R, U.S. Agency for Healthcare Research and Quality. *Quality of Care for General Medical Conditions: A Review of the Literature and Quality Indicators.* Santa Monica, CA: RAND Health; 2000.

54. Tregloan L. ISQua's 4th International Summit on Indicators, Buenos Aires, October 2001. *Int J Qual Health Care.* 2003;15(Suppl 1):i3–4.

55. Sunol R, Nicklin W, Bruneau C, Whittaker S. Promoting research into healthcare accreditation/external evaluation: advancing an ISQua initiative. *Int J Qual Health Care.* 2009;21(1):27–28.

56. Cerese J. Together we stand, collaborating we excel: partnering to target common goals. A report on and abstracts of the UHC (University HealthSystem Consortium) 2009 Quality and Safety Fall Forum. October 1–2, 2009. Atlanta, Georgia, USA. *Am J Med Qual.* 2010;25(2 Suppl):20S–36S.

57. Leapfrog Hospital Survey. 2011. Leapfrog Hospital Survey website. http://www .leapfroghospitalsurvey.org/. Accessed October 29, 2011.

58. Birkmeyer JD, Dimick JB. Potential benefits of the new Leapfrog standards: effect of process and outcomes measures. *Surgery.* 2004;135(6):569–575.

59. Brooke BS, Meguid RA, Makary MA, Perler BA, Pronovost PJ, Pawlik TM. Improving surgical outcomes through adoption of evidence-based process measures: intervention specific or associated with overall hospital quality? *Surgery.* 2010;147(4): 481–490.

60. DNV granted deeming authority from CMS. *Healthcare Benchmarks Qual Improv.* 2008;15(12):126–128.

61. Van Scyoc K. Process safety improvement—quality and target zero. *J Hazard Mater.* 2008;159(1):42–48.

62. About the 100 Top Hospitals Program. Thomson Reuters website. http://100top hospitals.com/about-100-top-hospitals/. Accessed April 9, 2012.

63. HealthGrades opening up methodology to review. *Healthcare Benchmarks Qual Improv.* 2004;11(8):89–90.

64. Comarow A. A look inside the hospital rankings. How 170 out of 5,453 centers made the cut. *U.S. News & World Report*. 2008;145(2):70, 72.

65. Kohn LCJ, Donaldson M. *To Err is Human: Building a Safer Health System*. National Academy Press; 2000.

66. Davenport DL, Holsapple CW, Conigliaro J. Assessing surgical quality using administrative and clinical data sets: a direct comparison of the University HealthSystem Consortium Clinical Database and the National Surgical Quality Improvement Program data set. *Am J Med Qual*. 2009;24(5):395–402.

67. Mack MJ, Herbert M, Prince S, Dewey TM, Magee MJ, Edgerton JR. Does reporting of coronary artery bypass grafting from administrative databases accurately reflect actual clinical outcomes? *J Thorac Cardiovasc Surg*. 2005;129(6):1309–1317.

68. Christian CK, Gustafson ML, Betensky RA, Daley J, Zinner MJ. The Leapfrog volume criteria may fall short in identifying high-quality surgical centers. *Ann Surg*. 2003;238(4):447–455; discussion 455-447.

69. Osborne NH, Ghaferi AA, Nicholas LH, Dimick JB. Evaluating popular media and Internet-based hospital quality ratings for cancer surgery. *Arch Surg*. 2011;146(5):600–604.

70. Osborne NH, Nicholas LH, Ghaferi AA, Upchurch GR, Jr., Dimick JB. Do popular media and Internet-based hospital quality ratings identify hospitals with better cardiovascular surgery outcomes? *J Am Coll Surg*. 2010;210(1):87–92.

71. Joseph B, Morton JM, Hernandez-Boussard T, Rubinfeld I, Faraj C, Velanovich V. Relationship between hospital volume, system clinical resources, and mortality in pancreatic resection. *J Am Coll Surg*. 2009;208(4):520–527.

72. Mansi IA, Shi R, Khan M, Huang J, Carden D. Effect of compliance with quality performance measures for heart failure on clinical outcomes in high-risk patients. *J Natl Med Assoc*. 2010;102(10):898–905.

73. Fonarow GC, Peterson ED. Heart failure performance measures and outcomes: real or illusory gains. *JAMA*. 2009;302(7):792–794.

Current State of Quality Measurement: Internal Dynamics

INTRODUCTION

There are many questions that have to be answered for quality efforts and initiatives to be successful. First, because health care is becoming increasingly evidence based, healthcare professionals expect to understand the rationale behind new initiatives and goals; that is, *what is the evidence?* Second, as the professional lives and work of these individuals revolve around direct patient care, what innovative means can be used to maintain focus and energy? Finally, how can individuals who are already highly regarded and highly paid for their skills be rewarded for outstanding performance? This chapter will answer these questions and introduce some methods that organizations use to meet performance targets.

GOALS AND OBJECTIVES

After reading this chapter, the reader should be able to:

1. Identify the healthcare priorities for an organization.
2. Discuss how organizations have mobilized to respond to quality improvement calls by involving their boards, management, and staffs.

3. Discuss the mandatory quality measures and how they are enforced.
4. Discuss the voluntary quality measures.
5. Discuss the need for a reliable measurement system that can be used to monitor progress toward targets and to generate reports.
6. Discuss the contents of a typical dashboard for quality.
7. Discuss the need for reporting and transparency.

HEALTHCARE QUALITY PRIORITIES: PATIENT SAFETY AND PATIENT EXPERIENCE

Healthcare professionals and students are well aware of the country's increasing healthcare costs. In 2010, healthcare spending accounted for 17.6% of the national GDP ($2.6 trillion) compared to 13.8% in 2000.[1,2] The United States spends more per capita on health care than any other country that is a member of the Organisation For Economic Co-operation and Development (OECD). In 2008, the United States spent an average of $7,538 per capita on health care, while Japan spent $2,729 per capita.[3] It is common knowledge that the U.S. healthcare system, although the most expensive, is not the most efficient. In 2010, the United States ranked last in The Commonwealth Fund's assessment of seven industrialized countries' health.[4] The public is becoming increasingly aware of the poor state of U.S. health system. Over 49 million Americans lack insurance, and of the Americans with health insurance, 9% are underinsured.[5,6] With 62% of bankruptcies related to medical care, Americans' concern for the system is justified.[7] According a Gallup poll, healthcare availability and affordability is rated as the fourth highest cause of concern, behind the economy, gas prices, and the federal budget.[8] As public dismay with the healthcare system swells, medical researchers themselves have come to a shocking realization. Not only is the American health system the world's most expensive, but it is also one of most dangerous healthcare systems in the world.

In 2000, the Institute of Medicine (IOM) published the groundbreaking report *To Err Is Human*, which brought international attention to the poor quality of American health care. According to the report, medical errors led to between 44,000 and 98,000 deaths per year in the United States. The estimated costs of increased medical bills and lost income ranged from $17 billion to $29 billion.

Although these estimates are shocking, it is important to note that some costs of poor-quality care such as the loss of a loved one and the pain of suffering with a reduced quality of life cannot be calculated.[9]

Although the report cited several potential causes of poor-quality care such as the fragmentation of the healthcare system or the complexity of payment systems, the report indicated that one reason for poor-quality care is inadequate performance-reporting procedures. An organization's or individual's fear of negative publicity or expensive litigation may encourage systems to administer poor performance reporting, which translates to poor problem detection, solution identification, and resolution.[10] The report provided several recommendations for the industry, government agencies, hospital systems, and healthcare providers. Healthcare leaders were invited to become more educated on the potential causes of error, the benefits of reporting of errors, and the science of setting of appropriate benchmarks. The report set the stage for a new era of healthcare quality and patient safety that would ultimately result in a new and improved patient experience.[9]

While the IOM definition of quality care encompasses six dimensions, the current focus on patient safety as the primary dimension potentially stems from the 2000 IOM publication of *To Err Is Human*,[9] which focused on and raised serious questions about patient safety in the context of general healthcare quality. Given the original Hippocratic Oath, which includes the commitment to *First, Do No Harm* as a guiding principle, these errors are unacceptable. There may well be other influencing factors; however, it does appear as though these have contributed to shaping the early debate on the quality of care in our healthcare system.

GOVERNANCE, MANAGEMENT, AND STAFF

Although certain kinds of initiatives can achieve success solely from "grass-roots" efforts, the achievement of high-level quality performance in healthcare organizations is not one of them. Attaining excellence in health care requires an unwavering commitment to quality from the very top of the organization. Without the visible commitment of the CEO and board, other senior and midlevel leaders will face difficulty gaining the "traction" required to improve quality.[11,12] This is a two-way street in the sense that if a healthcare organization has problems with quality, the problem starts at the very top of the organization. The Institute for Healthcare Improvement (IHI), the National Patient Safety Foundation, and other nonprofit and for-profit organizations can help make an effective case to raise awareness and obtain buy-in among the CEO and board of an organization.[13]

Hospitals and healthcare systems are complex organizations. Many different individuals play a role in the quality of care provided to patients and in the cost of care. Physicians, nurses, and pharmacists come to mind readily, but in reality there are countless technicians, allied health personnel, and clerical, administrative, supervisory, and executive staff who all have important roles. That said, physician actions are key to the quality and cost of care provided at hospitals, as physician decisions regarding diagnosis and treatment plans strongly influence the quality and drive most of the costs. Because physician reimbursement can take many forms, incentivizing physician commitment to quality initiatives may not be straightforward. Although the salaried workforce is employed, physicians may be associated with a hospital or health system in a variety of ways. Some may be salaried, some may be in independent private practice either as individuals or as members of a group, while others may be medical school faculty, and still others may be contracted to provide specific medical services, either individually or as a group. Therefore, motivating physicians and other groups of highly trained individuals to work toward common quality and financial goals can be a daunting task.

APPROACH TO QUALITY PRIORITIES

Organizations collect quality data for many reasons. Oftentimes, external factors require data collection and reporting. For example, the Centers for Medicare & Medicaid Services (CMS) and The Joint Commission (TJC) require submission of core measures data, which are increasingly public and which are used for reimbursement under Medicare's value-based purchasing (VBP) program. Other times, hospitals develop a desire to create custom quality metrics to monitor performance of a problem area or to assess the success of an initiative.

Mandatory Quality Data

The CMS core measures change yearly and are strongly evidence based, as most measures have been approved by the National Quality Forum (NQF). Although participation in core measures reporting has always been voluntary, CMS's partial withholding of payment for noncompliance made reporting essentially mandatory for nearly all U.S. hospitals. Because of the financial implications of nonreporting and the accompanying financial penalties, hospitals have little choice but to adopt CMS core measures as part of their internal quality reporting programs. Until the introduction of VBP by CMS (also known as Pay for Performance—P4P), hospitals did not have to reach any particular level of performance to receive full payment from CMS. With regard to service quality, for similar reasons hospitals are also obligated to report patient satisfaction data under the terms of CMS's Hospital Consumer Assessment of Healthcare Providers and Systems (HCAHPS). Again, until the advent of VBP, hospitals were not penalized for providing poor service quality. Hospitals and health systems may also be obligated to report certain quality, safety, and epidemiology measures to state and local governmental agencies.

Medicare's P4P programs, which will be used to adjust Medicare reimbursement rates, will also dictate the data collection and reporting procedures of hospitals. A 1% financial penalty for excessive readmissions of patients discharged after acute myocardial infarction, heart failure, and pneumonia will begin in 2013. This penalty applies to a hospital's entire payment for traditional Medicare patients, not just for patients in those three diagnostic groups. Five additional diagnostic groups will be added before 2015, when the readmission penalty escalates to a maximum of 3%. A new Medicare penalty of 1% will be applied in 2015 for hospitals in the upper quartile of all U.S. hospitals for the incidence of hospital-acquired conditions (HACs), which are also called "never events," because they should rarely if ever happen. Medicare-designated HACs are determined by diagnosis and procedure coding rules and include[14]:

- Vascular catheter-associated infections
- Catheter-associated urinary tract infections
- Pressure ulcers stages III and IV
- Blood incompatibility (transfusion reaction)
- Foreign object retained after surgery
- Air embolism
- Falls and trauma
- Manifestations of poor glycemic control
- Surgical site infection—mediastinitis after coronary artery bypass graft (CABG) procedures
- Surgical site infection after certain orthopedic procedures
- Surgical site infection after bariatric surgery for obesity
- Pulmonary embolism and deep venous thrombosis (DVT) for certain orthopedic procedures

CMS also requires hospitals to report multiple patient safety indicators (PSIs) endorsed by the NQF. PSIs are also determined by diagnosis and procedure coding rules. Some PSIs and HACs overlap in name, although they may be determined by different coding rules. Some NQF-endorsed PSIs include:

- Death in low-mortality diagnosis related groups (DRGs) (PSI 2)
- Decubitus ulcer (PSI 3)
- Death among surgical inpatients with serious treatable complications (PSI 4)
- Foreign body left during procedure, secondary diagnosis field (PSI 5)
- Iatrogenic pneumothorax, secondary diagnosis field (PSI 6)
- Selected infections due to medical care, secondary diagnosis field (PSI 7)
- Postoperative hip fracture (PSI 8)
- Postoperative respiratory failure (PSI 11)
- Postoperative pulmonary embolism or deep vein thrombosis (PSI 12)
- Postoperative sepsis (PSI 13)
- Postoperative wound dehiscence (PSI 14)
- Accidental puncture or laceration, secondary diagnosis field (PSI 15)
- Transfusion reaction, secondary diagnosis field (PSI 16 and 26)
- Birth trauma—injury to neonate (PSI 17)

The NQF has endorsed equivalent pediatric quality indicators (PDIs) as appropriate.

Beginning in 2012, CMS required acute-care hospitals to report central line–associated bloodstream infections (CLABSIs) to the Centers for Disease Control and Prevention (CDC) National Health Surveillance Network (NHSN) database registry. In 2013, certain types of surgical site infections (SSIs) must also be reported, along with catheter-associated urinary tract infections (CAUTIs). These hospital-acquired infections will likely become a component of VBP reimbursement in coming years.

Voluntary Quality Data

Hospitals and health systems may have elective, nonmandatory reasons for adoption of internal quality goals. Physicians, nurses, other caregivers, and administrators may have noted certain kinds of events that adversely affect patient care, such as medication or scheduling errors, and wish to decrease or eliminate them. Increasingly, such events must be reported to CMS or to state agencies, and the hospital may wish to address and control them at the earliest possible date before public reporting and penalties become mandatory.

Caregivers and administrators may wish to set goals for excellent patient care unrelated to national goals or any external reporting requirement. An example could be an operational improvement such as starting the operating room (OR) schedule on time or reducing the downtime between OR cases. Some internal goals can improve quality while simultaneously decreasing costs. For example, CLABSIs are associated with a 40% ICU mortality rate and approximately $35,000 in extra costs of care. Because of strong evidence that CLABSIs can be greatly reduced if not eliminated entirely with protocol-based catheter care, a hospital may wish to adopt a quality program independent of external reporting.[15,16]

Performance Requirements and Setting of Targets

After hospitals have set quality measures, they must set targets for performance. In doing so, it is important to keep the ultimate goal in sight because that is the only way it can be achieved. Because human lives are at stake, the ultimate goal for core measures compliance is 100%, and the ultimate goal for occurrence of adverse events such as HACs and PSIs is zero. Most core measures are process measures, and the linkage to better outcomes may not be obvious. However, there is growing evidence in the literature that process measure improvements have resulted in large-scale improvements in both survival and quality of life.[17–19] There will be those who believe that such high goals are unrealistic because all individuals make mistakes from time to time. Although that is certainly true, high-reliability organizations (HROs) such as those involved in air-traffic control, commercial aviation, naval aviation, nuclear submarines, and nuclear power have designed systems to ensure that human errors rarely if ever result in an accident or fatality. The U.S. nuclear submarine fleet has operated for more than 6,200 reactor-years of service without a single reactor accident as of March 2010.[20] Could that have occurred by chance? It has been argued that although humans may be expected to make errors from time to time, systems can be developed to ensure these errors are caught before they have a chance to produce harm.[21] Operating as an HRO has to be the ultimate goal for a healthcare organization in order to *First, Do No Harm*.[22,23] It should be noted that human beings are unlike items of machinery in that they may have many comorbidities and fatal conditions such as incurable cancer or irreversible heart failure and thus may have an unfavorable outcome in spite of the best of care. The importance of achieving core measures and avoiding adverse events remains undiminished as these patients will least tolerate any deviation from the highest quality of care.

There is another reason that hospitals should set very high goals. Organizations that perform at the 90% to 95% level on core measures will find it very hard to motivate caregivers and others to raise compliance another few percent.

Incremental goals are difficult to achieve, and in fact such efforts may never lead to 100% compliance. The difference between 95% performance and 100% performance is as important in health care as it is for air-traffic control or any other HRO. Most individuals would not fly on an airplane that had 95% of its servicing performed or live near a nuclear power plant where 95% of the safety checks were completed. There is a very large difference between the efforts required to reach 95% compliance with a quality measure and the efforts required to achieve 100%. To achieve 100%, work must be done differently, not just better, and multiple checks have to be put in place to ensure that lapses or errors fail to reach the patient. The "mindfulness" that an error may always occur is the prerequisite to ensuring that it does not.[24]

In a similar manner, the incidence of HACs and PSIs will never diminish if physicians, nurses, other caregivers, and administrators believe it is normal or acceptable for these events to occur. Every one of these events represents the equivalent of a mechanical failure in an airplane to the aviation industry or a reactor malfunction to the nuclear power industry. There is no "acceptable" level for these events to occur any more than there is an acceptable crash rate for an airline. This represents a major, maybe even difficult paradigm shift for many clinicians and administrators. Most senior clinicians and administrators began their careers long before these events were formally recorded, measured, and reported to federal and state governments. Additionally, the means and technology to prevent certain adverse events had not yet been discovered, even though the means may be as simple as a checklist or safety protocol. In a prior era, adverse events were considered "usual and customary" by-products of patient care.

The HACs and PSIs endorsed by the NQF are believed to be reasonably preventable if evidence-based care is provided. Therefore, the executive who sets goals for safety measures like HACs and PSIs must consider setting the goal at zero occurrences. It is very difficult to set targets for adverse events above zero when human lives are in the balance. However, if current performance is far short of the goal, an organization may wish to set an intermediate temporary target for a defined period of time. As the organization achieves the intermediate target, confidence is generated to go the rest of the distance. However, if an intermediate target is set above zero events of harm, it is important that everyone understand that the goal is always zero events.

One method of improving performance is to set internal goals such that on a monthly basis, only 100% performance for each quality measure is rewarded, and only zero occurrence of each HAC and PSI is rewarded. Each facility or clinical unit has a fresh chance at perfect performance each month, so the goal is set in terms of the number of months each measure is at 100% compliance with zero occurrence of harmful events, as appropriate.

Implementation of Reliable Measurement Systems

Clinical care processes can be difficult to measure. Caregivers have little time for extra measurements, paperwork, and computer data entry. However, the saying "You can't manage what you don't measure" is perhaps more true for health care than it is for other industries. At present, most data for quality measurements are gathered in two ways, although a third method is about to supervene. The first method is clinical chart abstraction in which trained human abstractors, typically nurses, review charts to determine if core measures were met. Abstractors not only look for evidence that a core measure was achieved by providing a timely medication or other treatment, but they also review the chart for documentation of valid exception conditions when a medication or treatment could not reasonably be given, perhaps due to a preexisting drug allergy. If a valid exception or contraindication has been documented by a physician, the core measure is considered compliant. The second way quality is extracted from a chart is from the coding of diagnoses and procedures. This also requires human chart abstraction, but with a different set of individuals charged with abstracting the most appropriate diagnosis, procedure, and billing codes. In most states, each diagnosis must be marked as either present on admission (POA) or not present on admission (non-POA), which makes it possible for coding rules to determine when a condition, such as an infection, is hospital acquired.

The most reliable way to enable caregivers to record quality data is to make it part of their normal workflow. Many quality-related parameters, such as the time of medication administration, can be automatically extracted from an electronic chart. That is the basis for the abstraction method that will supervene over the next few years—extraction of quality data from an electronic health record (EHR), in compliance with "meaningful use" requirements from the American Recovery and Reinvestment Act (ARRA) of 2009. *Meaningful use* refers to ARRA's requirement that hospitals report an increasing amount of quality data to CMS electronically and without after-the-fact human abstraction. This represents a very major change in workflow because it means that the data needed to adjudicate core measures compliance has to be in coded form in the electronic chart rather than in handwritten or transcribed notes.[25]

In any case, performance cannot be improved unless it is measured, and there is no way to know if performance has improved or degraded without measurement. If a surgical safety checklist is implemented to ensure the safety of patients undergoing surgery, then compliance with actual use of the checklist must be measured.[26,27] If safety "bundles" are implemented to ensure sterile insertion and maintenance of central venous catheters, then compliance with the bundles has to be measured. Implementation of quality process measures without assessment of compliance is an empty gesture not likely to be effective in improvement of patient care. Indeed, quality process measures are frequently reported as compliance rates. The challenge is to incorporate the measurement into the care and documentation process such that it is part of the normal workflow. As an example, elements of the central line bundle can be incorporated into the EHR, which allows the data to be automatically extracted later. The EHR serves two important purposes: (1) it provides the user with a safety bundle checklist to guide the procedure, and (2) it provides a coded record that can be extracted to produce compliance measurements for each element of the bundle.

Achieving Transparency for Results

The finest quality measurements will have no impact if they are not published in a timely fashion. The nature of clinical care is that it is fast moving. The events of 3 and 6 months ago are a distant memory to most caregivers and replaced with consideration of more recent patients and events. Therefore, the key is to relay results back to caregivers and others who can make a difference in the shortest possible time and at a frequency that allows for rapid cycle improvement. Measurements more than a month old are useful only for summary purposes rather than as a basis for action. The challenge is to reduce the report production interval and to get results in front of users monthly if not more frequently. In addition, paper reports are costly to produce and distribute and may be prone to inadvertent disclosure if a report is accidentally left in a public venue.

PERFORMANCE DASHBOARDS

Different types of dashboards are needed for different parts and levels of the healthcare organization. For direct caregiver clinical care improvements, dashboards may be needed at the hospital, department, and care unit levels. Executives need summarized dashboards with drill-down capability to identify high- and low-performing units. Highly summarized dashboards are required for use at higher levels of the organization. The board of directors reviews performance from many different areas of the healthcare organization, and for that reason a more highly summarized dashboard is required for their use.

REFERENCES

1. Flemming C. U.S. health spending projected to grow 5.8 percent annually. Health Affairs Blog website. http://healthaffairs.org/blog/2011/07/28/u-s-health-spending-projected-to-grow-5-8-percent-annually/. Accessed April 3, 2012.

2. Centers for Medicare & Medicaid Services. NHE summary including share of GDP, CY 1960–2010; Historical National Health Expenditure Data. CMS website. http://www.cms.gov/Research-Statistics-Data-and-Systems/Statistics-Trends-and-Reports/NationalHealthExpendData/NationalHealthAccountsHistorical.html. Accessed April 9, 2012.

3. Health Care Market Place Project. Snapshots: health care spending in the United States and selected OECD countries, April 2011. Kaiser Family Foundation website. http://www.kff.org/insurance/snapshot/oecd042111.cfm. Accessed April 3, 2012.

4. Davis K, Schoen C, Stremikis K. Mirror, Mirror on the Wall: How the Performance of the U.S. Health Care System Compares Internationally, 2010 Update. The Commonwealth Fund, June 2010.

5. Schoen C, Collins SR, Kriss JL, Doty MM. How many are underinsured? Trends among U.S. adults, 2003 and 2007. *Health Affairs* Web Exclusive, June 10, 2008, w298–w309.

6. Les C. Number of people without health insurance climbs. CNN Money website. http://money.cnn.com/2011/09/13/news/economy/census_bureau_health_insurance/index.htm. Accessed April 3, 2012.

7. Himmelstein DU, Thorne D, Warren E, Woolhandler S. Medical bankruptcy in the United States, 2007: results of a national study. *Am J Med.* 2009;122:741–746.

8. Saad L. Economic issues still dominate Americans' national worries. Gallup website. http://www.gallup.com/poll/153485/Economic-Issues-Dominate-Americans-National-Worries.aspx. Accessed April 3, 2012.

9. Kohn LCJ, Donaldson M. *To Err is Human: Building a Safer Health System.* Washington, DC: National Academy Press; 2000.

10. Leape LL, Brennan TA, Laird N, et al. The nature of adverse events in hospitalized patients. Results of the Harvard Medical Practice Study II. *N Engl J Med.* 1991;324(6):377–384.

11. Jha A, Epstein A. Hospital governance and the quality of care. *Health Aff (Millwood).* 2010;29(1):182–187.

12. Vaughn T, Koepke M, Kroch E, Lehrman W, Sinha S, Levey S. Engagement of leadership in quality improvement initiatives: executive quality improvement survey results. *J Patient Saf.* 2006;2(1):2–9.

13. 5 Million Lives Campaign. Getting started kit: Governance leadership "boards on board" how-to guide. Institute for Healthcare Improvement website. http://www.ihi.org/knowledge/Pages/Tools/HowtoGuideGovernanceLeadership.aspx. Accessed November 6, 2011.

14. Hospital-acquired conditions. Centers for Medicare & Medicaid Services website. https://www.cms.gov/hospitalacqcond/06_hospital-acquired_conditions.asp. Accessed December 15, 2011.

15. Clancy CM. The canary's warning: why infections matter. *Am J Med Qual.* 2009;24(6):462–464.

16. Pronovost P, Needham D, Berenholtz S, et al. An intervention to decrease catheter-related bloodstream infections in the ICU. *N Engl J Med.* 2006;355(26):2725–2732.

17. Hospital deaths from heart failure cut by half over seven years. *AHRQ News and Numbers*. http://www.ahrq.gov/news/nn/nn082511.htm. Published August 25, 2011. Accessed November 21, 2011.

18. Chassin MR, Loeb JM, Schmaltz SP, Wachter RM. Accountability measures— using measurement to promote quality improvement. *N Engl J Med*. 2010;363(7): 683–688.

19. Krumholz HM, Wang Y, Chen J, et al. Reduction in acute myocardial infarction mortality in the United States: risk-standardized mortality rates from 1995–2006. *JAMA*. 2009;302(7):767–773.

20. Nuclear-powered ships. World Nuclear Association website. http://www.world -nuclear.org/info/inf34.html. Published 2011. Accessed December 15, 2011.

21. Reason J. Human error: models and management. *BMJ*. 2000;320(7237):768–770.

22. Chassin MR, Loeb JM. The ongoing quality improvement journey: next stop, high reliability. *Health Aff (Millwood)*. 2011;30(4):559–568.

23. Wolterman D, Shabot MM. A new standard. Aim for safety of planes, nuclear plants. *Mod Healthc*. 2011;41(31):27.

24. Weick KE, Sutcliffe KM. *Managing the Unexpected: Assuring High Performance in an Age of Complexity*. San Francisco, CA: Jossey-Bass; 2001.

25. Bria WF, 2nd, Shabot MM. The electronic medical record, safety, and critical care. *Crit Care Clin*. 2005;21(1):55–79, viii.

26. Gawande A. *The Checklist Manifesto: How to Get Things Right*. New York, NY: Metropolitan Books; 2010.

27. Haynes AB, Weiser TG, Berry WR, et al. A surgical safety checklist to reduce morbidity and mortality in a global population. *N Engl J Med*. 2009;360(5):491–499.

Measuring Quality of Inpatient Care

INTRODUCTION

In order for a healthcare organization to be in control of the quality of care it delivers, a carefully designed performance measurement and reporting system is required. It is important to separate the questions of what to measure and how to handle the measured performance. The former has to do with the appropriateness of the performance measure itself, whereas the latter addresses data management and processing. It is this latter component that requires a well-crafted framework. The requirement for the performance measure would be to find its appropriate placement within the framework. This chapter presents a framework for the measurement of healthcare quality with a primary focus on inpatient care. This framework is intended to provide a basis for healthcare providers operationally to define, measure, report, monitor, and improve quality of care in a way that can meaningfully be addressed at multiple levels within the provider organization. The related literature and logical construct and backbone of this framework are also discussed.

GOALS AND OBJECTIVES

After reading this chapter, the reader should be able to:

1. Define quality in health care and discuss its domains and dimensions.
2. Define the terms *measure*, *indicator*, and *metric*.

3. Discuss the role of outcome in assessment of quality performance.
4. Discuss the attributes of a quality performance measure.
5. Discuss the components of a comprehensive performance measurement framework.
6. Discuss scoring and aggregation schemas for a performance measurement framework.

BEFORE THE MEASUREMENT PROCESS BEGINS

Earlier in this text, it was argued that the current approach to quality of care by the organizations that have taken leadership roles in this area is not encompassing of the full scope and definition of quality of care. At the same time, healthcare organizations have all but surrendered to the proposed methods and measures of these organizations, such as the core measures of The Joint Commission (TJC; formerly the Joint Commission on Accreditation of Healthcare Organizations, or JCAHO). For an organization to truly deliver high-quality care, it must reexamine the concepts associated with quality in health care and more carefully translate those concepts into practical and consistent approaches to measurement, reportage, and improvement of quality.

This reexamination should start with a clear philosophy of measurement. Measurement is conducted for various reasons; however, one reason dominates all else when it comes to measurement of quality in any industry including health care, and that is to be able to make changes and improve quality. Solely measuring outcomes, although they arguably are the closest surrogate for quality of care, is not very helpful as it does not readily offer insight into the changes required to improve the outcomes. Therefore, other modifiable variables that can affect the outcomes must be identified and measured. Many of these variables are part of the *process* of care.

Given that measurement is necessary, significant questions such as what and how to measure should be addressed. Before addressing these questions, a deeper understanding of the context of quality of care is also necessary. Although healthcare services are delivered in various contexts, the focus of this text is on hospitals and inpatient care. Consequently, the characteristics of this context and how inpatient care fits into the continuum of care should be examined. For example, an often relied-on quality measure and a TJC core measure is "smoking cessation counseling." In fact, the hospital has little control over whether patients stop smoking. Patients will make that decision on their own after discharge. Thus, it is not clear whether such a recommendation would change the outcome at the time of discharge from a hospital, whether patients will stop smoking, or whether the final outcome will result in fewer deaths or repeat heart attacks.[1] Whereas it is good medical practice to advise all patients to stop smoking, having this advice as a measure of quality of care for a hospital is outside the inpatient context of care and seemingly irrelevant to judging the quality of inpatient care. A more appropriate context for this advice to patients would be the follow-up primary care or physician office visit after hospitalization, where patient compliance with postdischarge medical advice could be measured.

Reliance on administrative data to determine quality of care in a healthcare system or hospital may well be limited by questions of data consistency and quality and by a lack of depth and clinical insight into the process of care.[2,3]

Effective measurement of care quality in a hospital requires careful examination and documentation of procedures and processes. Root-cause analyses of failures in the past and examination of workflow and patient flow, including all steps from admission to discharge, would help identify the key processes in the delivery of care. These procedures and processes can then be translated into quality measures. An effective healthcare quality measurement system should allow for an observed change in outcome to be traced back to the causative factors in a way that then guides specific process changes that will improve outcomes. Any healthcare organization committed to improving its quality of care should monitor, record, and report its outcomes. Process measures that are linked to outcomes and can allow processes to be adjusted to improve overall outcomes, and thus quality, are essential to the functioning of hospital organizations (and, in general, providers). However, other stakeholders may not share the same level of interest in process measures. In fact, it will better serve payers and policy stakeholders to move their focus to outcomes and transition from process measures that at best may not translate to improved outcomes and at worst may be manipulated to increase reimbursement.

DEFINITION OF HEALTHCARE QUALITY

A review of the history of healthcare quality was previously presented in this text, followed by a review of the current landscape in healthcare quality that listed a number of prominent organizations that are active in this field. In a very general sense, these organizations have the goal of improving quality in healthcare delivery. Having discussed the dependence of quality improvement on quality measurement, it becomes clear that a definition for healthcare quality is needed to clarify what is to be measured. The Institute of Medicine (IOM) definition for quality of health care was offered earlier in this text as a broad and workable definition that can be used by all parties involved in the continuum that makes up the healthcare system. This text will adopt the IOM definition as the basis for the concepts that will be presented. The IOM defines healthcare quality as[4,5]:

> The degree to which health services for individuals and populations increase the likelihood of desired health outcomes and are consistent with current professional knowledge.

This definition is followed by six aims put forth by the IOM to focus efforts for improvement of quality. These aims are safety, effectiveness, patient centeredness, timeliness, efficiency, and equitability.[2]

TERMINOLOGY

For the purpose of this text, the following definitions will be used. A quality measure is defined as "a mechanism to assign a quantity to quality of care by comparison to a criterion."[6] This definition is expanded to define a performance measure as a mechanism to assign a quantity to a variable of interest according to a criterion within the context of care and related to the quality of care as defined by the IOM.

A performance indicator is defined as a composite of measures grouped together according to a consensus on the part of the organization. Subsequently, a quality indicator is defined as a composite of quality measures that represent a specific dimension (or domain) of quality for a specific function or operation within the organization. In the context of this text, different dimensions of healthcare quality are grouped under six main categories represented by the six aims (dimensions) introduced by IOM. Therefore, there will be six groups of quality indicators. Finally, a performance metric is defined as a summary representation of a group of indicators that are closely related to a broad aspect of organizational performance, such as finance and quality. A quality metric represents performance under one or more quality dimensions for a group of functions or operations within the organization (**Figure 6-1**).

For example, the labeling of medication bags with a patient's name and medical record number is a quality measure that deals with the medication safety dimension of quality. This labeling can be grouped with other measures of medication safety to produce a medication safety indicator, which will be listed under safety, one of the

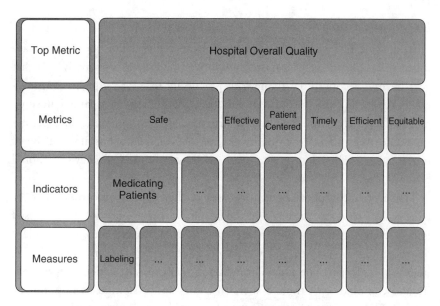

FIGURE 6-1. A hierarchical view of quality measures, indicators, and metrics. Metrics correspond to one or more of the IOM aims. An organization can create an aggregate value of the metrics as "top quality metric" and define it as appropriate to represent the organization's quality performance level. Of course, boundaries have to be defined, and the metric must have true meaning. This will allow an organization periodically to monitor its performance with respect to quality.

six aims of the IOM mentioned previously. Eventually, safety indicators separately or in conjunction with other indicators for the other five aims can be used to make up a quality metric that addresses only safety or a larger group of quality aims.

MEASUREMENT FRAMEWORK

An effective process for measurement of quality is dependent on having a conceptual framework that incorporates the issues raised in the previous section "Before the Measurement Process Begins."

This framework should also be based on an accepted working definition for quality in health care. At this point, the IOM definition with its six aims appears to be the most complete and most appropriate foundation upon which to build a measurement system. In the following paragraphs, a framework for measurement of quality of health care is outlined, and emphasis is placed on inpatient care in a hospital setting. Figure 6-1 shows the outline of this framework.

Define the Context

First, the specific environmental *context* for care delivery must be clearly established to ensure the development of an operational measurement system that goes beyond a conceptual framework practically to address quality improvement. Again, for the purposes of this text, the context is inpatient hospital medical care. Therefore, any access, structure, process, outcome, and patient experience that affects the quality of care delivered in a hospital will be of interest. For other contexts (i.e., care settings), a similar framework should be developed.

However, a complicating factor arises in that certain outcomes could be affected by processes that begin in the hospital context, but the outcome itself is not solely or entirely within the context of a hospital and is dependent on continuity of care to and within other contexts (e.g., ambulatory care, home care). To this one must also add considerations of patient responsibility and compliance. Although such outcomes are of significant importance, ultimately they are measures of quality for the larger healthcare delivery system, and the hospital can only be accountable for the processes at the time of discharge. These processes are necessary but not sufficient to secure the expected outcomes.

Processes that fall outside of the hospital inpatient context include such things as smoking cessation counseling, mentioned earlier. Although it is important to ensure that best practices associated with these non-inpatient care processes are followed, such processes (outside the true inpatient arena) are not reflective of the quality of care delivered in the hospital inpatient context. And unless all patients upon discharge are tracked for outcomes after discharge, the mere initiation of such processes on the part of the hospital would not necessarily result in a measurable improvement in quality as determined by an improvement in outcomes.

Consequently, measuring or judging the quality of hospital inpatient care by the presence/initiation of such processes is questionable. To build on the smoking cessation example, it is true that smoking contributes to increased risk of stroke and heart attack. It is also true that patients that stop smoking will gradually reduce their risk of stroke and heart attacks. However, the association between smoking cessation counseling upon discharge in reducing the risk of adverse outcomes is far less clear, and therefore measurement of such practices (processes) is not an appropriate measurement of inpatient quality of care.[1] In fact, Medicare is now moving away from process measures for determination of quality and is shifting attention to outcome measures.[7]

Define Organizational Operations and Create Related Groups

Second, the services delivered—organizational operations performed—in the appropriate context should be defined such that there is a trigger, or beginning, and a conclusion, or ending, for each of them. There are thousands of organizational operations in a particular context, and each will depend on access, structures, and processes that support them and will result in patient experience, and outcomes that may need improvement. These operations should then be grouped according to the general functions of the context in question. For instance, a hospital organization is a place where medical problems, or conditions, are diagnosed and treated—using medications or invasive interventions—by medical staff relying on the support services available to the hospital, either internally or externally. Therefore, one may classify the operations within a hospital into three classes or categories:

1. Medical conditions that require evaluation and workup until a diagnosis is made. These will be referred to as *diagnoses*; for example, heart attack, or myocardial infarction, where diagnosis begins when a patient with chest pain presents to the emergency department and concludes when the patient is rolled into a catheterization laboratory for intervention.

2. Invasive interventions that are required either to treat or manage a patient with a diagnosis or are needed to establish a diagnosis and are part of the workup of a patient. These will be referred to as *interventions*; for example, surgical intervention for acute cholecystitis, which begins when a diagnosis is made and concludes when the patient is discharged.

3. Laboratory tests, imaging studies, pharmacy, and so forth that participate in the process of diagnosis or management of a patient. These will be referred to as *services*; for example, computerized tomography (CT scan) for stroke, which begins when a CT is ordered by a medical professional and concludes when a report is submitted by a radiologist.

Link Operational Categories to the IOM Aims

Third, each of the described classes or categories should be evaluated with respect to the six IOM aims. The data required for each of the aims will come from measures for each operation under a class or category.

Link Operational Measures to Access, Structure, Process, Outcome, and Patient Experience

Fourth, operations under each of the described classes or categories will involve the five domains of access, structure, process, outcome, and patient experience.

To improve the outcome, the operation's access, structure, process, and patient experience must be carefully studied. It is noteworthy that process measures can be determined in real time whereas outcome measures usually cannot. For instance, using computerized physician order entry (CPOE), the information about how quickly antibiotics were ordered for a patient with pneumonia is available as soon as the order is entered. However, the outcome of this order, whether it is the time when the patient actually received the antibiotic (if the medication administration record [MAR] is paper based) or if the patient improved with the antibiotic, may not be available immediately. Structure measures are static and will change as a result of reorganization. Access is an important determinant of outcome. Whether certain interventions or tests or other healthcare services are available to a patient can significantly influence the outcome of care. However, in the context of an operation, access is a binary variable—the patient either has access to the operation or does not. Patient experience is often an after-the-fact measure and not only may influence the outcome but may also be influenced by the outcome. Access precedes the operation, and patient experience spans the full scope of the operation (**Figure 6-2**). Finally, in this framework, outcome—or the result—from one operation may become part of the input to another operation

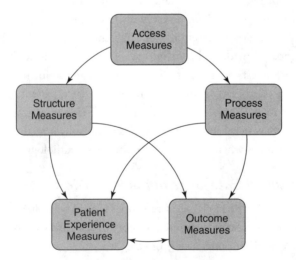

FIGURE 6-2. The relationship among quality measures in each of the modified Donabedian domains of quality. Most relationships are unidirectional, meaning one domain may influence another domain but not be influenced by it; however, outcome and patient experience domains may have a bidirectional relationship.

and will therefore have an effect on that other operation. Such outcomes may be used as process measures for another operation.

Link Operational Measures to the IOM Aims

Fifth, quality measures identified for each of the operations will be evaluated to determine their contribution to each of the six aims, recognizing that one measure may contribute to more than one aim. Additionally, one operation's quality measure will not necessarily contribute to all six aims.

As discussed earlier, an operation's outcome may also function as a process measure for another operation. An outcome measure from one operation, operation A, may only serve as a process measure in another operation, operation B; clearly, operation B will have outcome measures of its own. Operations A and B may not necessarily be under the same category or class in a context. Finally, a measure from operation A that also serves as a measure in operation B may affect different IOM aims for operation A than for operation B. The following example helps clarify these concepts.

Consider a hospital where initiation of treatment for stroke (operation B, *interventions* category) is slower than that by local competition. Assume that this is the result of a delay in the diagnosis of nonhemorrhagic stroke, which in turn is due to the delay in the availability of the imaging report (operation A, *services* category). In this case, the outcome in imaging (operation A outcome: time from order to report) in the services category of hospital operations is the cause of a deficiency in timeliness in the interventions category of the hospital's operations. The same outcome measure, which also serves as a process measure for operation B (i.e., interventions for stroke), will adversely affect the timeliness of care, as well as the effectiveness of care in the interventions category, and will also adversely affect the timeliness of the services category. This problem may be traced to a structural deficiency, which is the geographical distance of the imaging equipment from the emergency department. A solution could be the installation of dedicated imaging equipment in the emergency department.

Case-Mix and Other Context-Specific Considerations

Sixth, when collecting data and preparing aggregate numbers—indicators and metrics—for IOM aims, consideration must be given to the specific patient population that the hospital organization serves. The aggregate numbers must represent the frequency of different diagnoses, interventions, or services as well as severity of medical diagnoses or complexity of interventions. This is also referred to as risk adjustment or case-mix (equivalent to input variation in manufacturing).

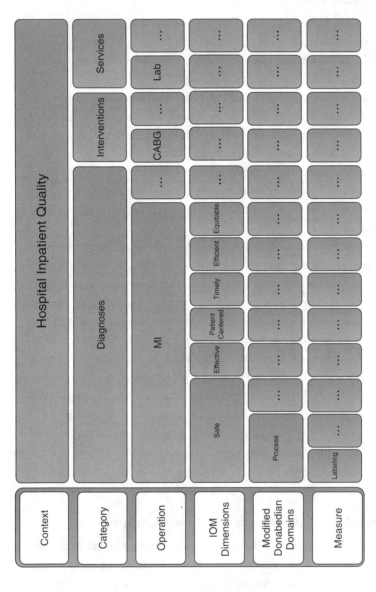

FIGURE 6-3. A depiction of the quality measurement framework. At the top, the context must be identified. This is followed by categories of operations and then a listing of operations under each category. The six IOM aims will be evaluated for each operation. Under each aim, access, structure, process, outcome, and patient experience will be examined. In the end, measures are defined. The setup for metrics, indicators, and measures was discussed earlier and requires case-mix considerations as well as weighting according to the frequency of operations in each category. MI, myocardial infarction; CABG, coronary artery bypass graft; Admin. techn., administration technique.

Figure 6-3 captures the placement of context, categories of operations, and the six IOM aims in this framework. Principles of this framework could also be used for other healthcare contexts, such as ambulatory care or rehabilitation care, with minimal modifications mainly to classes or categories of operations.

QUALITY MEASURES

A quality measure is a mechanism that enables the user to quantify a selected aspect of care by comparing it to a criterion.[6] The selected aspect of care can be outcome, financial efficiency, or clinical performance. The result of this comparison can have internal and external implications for any user, including a hospital organization, which is the focus of this discussion. The internal use would be to create methods to improve the quality of care in the hospital, and the external use would be to compare the quality performance of a hospital to that of another hospital.[8]

Measures can have specific focus areas; for example, a clinical performance measure can be viewed as a mechanism for assessing the degree to which a provider competently and safely delivers clinical services that are appropriate for the patient in the optimal time period.[9,10] This can be expanded to include characteristics of health care along all of the six aims introduced by IOM.

The National Quality Measures Clearinghouse (NQMC), which is sponsored by the Agency for Healthcare Research and Quality (AHRQ), provides information on how to develop a quality measure and has described five domains of interest, each of which offers a different insight into healthcare quality.[11] These are as follows:

1. Access: assesses the patient's attainment of timely and appropriate health care.
2. Structure: a feature of a healthcare organization or clinician relevant to its capacity to provide health care.
3. Process: assesses a healthcare service provided to, or on behalf of, a patient.
4. Outcome: the health state of a patient resulting from health care.
5. Patient experience: aggregates the reports of patients about their observations of and participation in health care.

According to the NQMC, the desirable attributes of a measure can be grouped into three concept areas within which narrower categories provide more detail[12]:

1. Importance of the Measure
   a. *Relevance to stakeholders.* The measure is of significant interest and is financially and strategically important to stakeholders (i.e., businesses, clinicians, and patients).

    b. *Health importance.* The measure addresses a clinically important aspect of health as defined by high prevalence or incidence and has a significant effect on the burden of illness (i.e., mortality and morbidity).

    c. *Applicable to measuring the equitable distribution of health care.* The measure can be used to examine whether disparities in care exist among different patient populations.

    d. *Potential for improvement.* Variations of quality among organizations necessitate quality improvement and process monitoring.

    e. *Susceptibility to being influenced by the healthcare system.* Actions or interventions based on the measure lead to improvements in quality.

2. Scientific Soundness

    a. *Clinical logic.* Must be reasonable and rational.

    b. *Explicitness of evidence.* There must be supporting evidence for the measure.

    c. *Strength of evidence.* The measure must have impact in its clinical area.

    d. *Measure properties.* The characteristics of the measure must be clearly defined.

    e. *Reliability.* The measure results should be reproducible and reflect results of actions implemented over time. Reliability testing should also be documented.

    f. *Validity.* The measure should in fact measure what it purports to measure. Validity testing should be documented.

    g. *Allowance for patient and consumer factors.* The measure should accommodate stratification or case-mix adjustment.

    h. *Comprehensible.* The results of the measure should be understandable for the users of the data.

3. Feasibility

    a. *Explicit specification of numerator and denominator.* The numerator and denominator for the measure should be clearly defined, and data collection should be possible.

    b. *Data availability.* The data for the measure should be available, accessible, timely, and cost effective.

OPERATIONALIZING THE MEASUREMENT FRAMEWORK

Once measures are identified, they can be quantified. The numerical values assigned to these measures will have different units and scales and will not be comparable. For example, some measures may be represented in minutes, whereas others are represented in a generic scale and yet others may be binary. As a result of different units of measurement, aggregating them to form indicators, and eventually metrics, will be impossible. One way to address this difficulty would be to use a consistent scoring system for measures. To have a scoring system that allows aggregation of measures into indicators and indicators into metrics, certain conditions must be satisfied.

As discussed earlier in the section "Measurement Framework," this framework for quality measurement requires a well-defined operation with a clear beginning and ending. Within that operation, access, structure, process, and outcome as well as patient experience measures should be defined. Clearly, a healthcare organization cannot keep track of all measures all of the time. There should be a sampling scheme that allows the organization to monitor quality of care. To appreciate the impact of a structure, process, or patient experience measure on any sample case that represents an operation, the analysis of measurements should be done when the operation is complete. Access should be evaluated as the percentage of patients who meet the medical indication for the represented operation and are eligible to have the operation safely and in fact receive it. Once a sufficient number of such case studies are complete, the organization should have a reasonable understanding of the significance and behavior of the access, structure, process, or patient experience measure on the outcomes of the operation. As appropriate, this could lead to real-time gathering of data and monitoring of the measures.

To have meaningful scores that do not change upward and downward over time as a result of a change in organizational, regional, or national averages, each score must describe an absolute condition that is incrementally superior to the one below it and incrementally inferior to the one above it. For example, if a measure is described as "above average" or "within top five percent" as the organization—or the industry for that matter—improves the quality of care it delivers, the average or top five percent range changes, and it becomes harder to rank measures in that category.

Another requirement is that the scores describe the measure in terms of its effect on the dimension it describes independently of the dimension. In other words, all six IOM aims (dimentions) should have the same scoring scheme within the framework. As a result of this consistency, scores could be better understood by the stakeholders (managers, executives, board members, and even patients). One way to accomplish this would be to grade the measures according to the consequences of the deficiency in performance. For example, if having zero deficiencies is the ideal score, it will define a performance that meets the specifications completely and is associated with no adverse outcome. The next best score will perhaps be zero deficiencies of consequence, underlining the fact that no deficiencies were linked to an adverse outcome. These associations can only be known when the operation is complete. As mentioned before, when sufficient numbers of sampled cases are studied, the numerical values of measures can be statistically linked to scores within a confidence interval. When the organization reaches this point, real-time monitoring of quality measures becomes possible. Even then, ongoing sampling is necessary to keep track of changes in performance and to maintain validity and reliability of the scoring system.

Quality measurement cannot be expected to run on autopilot. This may sound redundant, but it underlines the fact that the setup and implementation of a quality monitoring system takes time and effort. It should be customized and tailored to the organization.

Therefore, at least until the system is completely integrated with the organization's operations and validity and reliability of measures are ascertained, every sampled case must be carefully examined and its measures and outcomes carefully correlated. Such a scoring system is superior to the measurement of compliance with the requirements in that it links the measure to an outcome and provides gradations of performance that although not perfect, result in no change in the outcome. For example, compliance with administration of antibiotics with a certain time for diagnoses of pneumonia may increase as a result of over-diagnosis of pneumonia. This is inefficient. However, reporting this performance measure in terms of deficiencies as shown in **Figure 6-4** will remove the incentive to over treat and can accurately determine whether

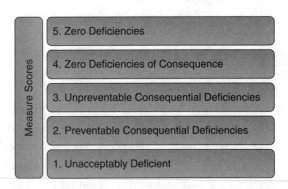

FIGURE 6-4. A scoring scheme with five levels, with 5 being the best score.

to link this measure to the outcome, which is clearly lacking in mere reporting of compliance.

One such scoring system that offers five levels is presented in Figure 6-4. An example of putting a quality measure in such a system would be the case of surgical wound infection. A process measure, for example, surgical site care, can be scored in terms of its success in controlling infection as a score of two, meaning there are preventable and consequential deficiencies as seen in the rate of infections. This is more understandable and useful than knowing that 92% of surgeries were compliant with the requirements of the surgical site care measure. As will be seen later, this also makes aggregation of measures into indicators and metrics possible.

Compiling Raw Measure Data into Meaningful Information

The framework presented in this chapter provides a basic depiction of the various moving elements of the quality domains and dimensions of care. Assigning a score to a measure is only the first step in analyzing the quality of care data. It is necessary to use constructs that could point out performance information in each domain and dimension so corrective action could take place in the case of a deficiency. Additionally, such a construct could also highlight areas of vulnerability within the system that could jeopardize the outcomes. For example, a healthcare system may still have acceptable or superior outcomes even in the face of deficiencies in the process or structure through compensatory actions by the clinicians or other compensating factors. This situation is far from robust, and having information about all of the domains of quality will provide grounds for corrective and preventive action.

A logical approach to compiling the raw measure scores into usable information is discussed here. Although this approach may appear overly complex, it must be emphasized that in practice, the number of measures defined for each operation will be limited, and therefore these calculations will be simpler and more manageable.

First, a sample of the operation must be taken and all the measures scored with respect to a standard scoring system, such as the one in Figure 6-4. Building on the example of surgical site care, if 6 out of 25 surgery cases sampled have developed a preventable infection, then, this measure is scored at 2.

It is important to understand that outcomes are the end product of the operation, but they still can be scored the same way as other measures. The operation is defined within a clinical context. This may become confusing for operations in the support services category because every time a test is performed, a result is produced, and the rates of deficiencies may be extremely low. However, the operation for a support service starts when the order is placed and ends when the report is filed. Whether the outcome was deficient should be judged by whether the report addressed the reason the service was requested or whether the report arrived when it was expected.

Using the framework presented in Figure 6-3, one could aggregate the measures across the domains or IOM aims (dimentions). Although both approaches have merits, it may be more useful to aggregate the measures across the six IOM aims as they provide more understandable quality reports. During the planning process, thinking about the domains may provide a deeper insight into solutions for a corrective approach; however, the measures by themselves will be more useful than aggregates across the five domains.

Aggregation of Measures into Indicators for Each Operation

To produce quality indicators that correspond to the six IOM aims for each operation, first each measure must be assigned a weight that reflects the impact of the measure on the quality dimension. As shown in **Figure 6-5**, the strength of correlation between the measure and the aim may be strong, minimal, or somewhere in between. To ensure consistency of results with the scoring system, the highest correlation will be shown as 1 and the weakest as 0. In the following paragraphs, the mechanisms are formalized using mathematical notations.

To aggregate the measures for an operation into an indicator for that operation in one of the IOM aims, a weighted averaging method such as shown in **Equation 6-1** could be used. This approach ensures that the strength of

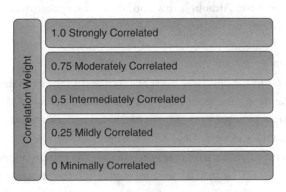

FIGURE 6-5. Assigning a weight to the magnitude of effect a quality measure has on an IOM aim in a given operation.

correlation (shown in Figure 6-5) between the measure and the outcome of the operation is considered.

$$I_a^0 = \frac{\sum_{i=0}^{n} R^{o,a} \cdot m_i^o}{\sum_{i=0}^{n} R^{o,a}}$$

Equation 6-1. Calculation of indicator I for operation o and IOM aim a. $R^{o,a}$ represents the correlation weight (range 0–1) for measure m_i^o to IOM aim a.

Similarly, indicators for each of the five domains of access, structure, process, outcome, and patient experience can be calculated for each operation, only in this case there is no correlation weight as the correlation weight for a measure in a domain on the indicator for that domain will simply be 1 (**Equation 6-2**). Therefore, simple averaging will produce the indicator.

$$I_d^o = \frac{\sum_{i=o}^{n} m_{d,i}}{n}$$

Equation 6-2. Calculation of indicator I for domain d in operation o.

Aggregation of Indicators into Metrics for Operational Categories

Using a similar logic for the calculation of indicators from measures, IOM indicators for each operation can be used to calculate the metrics for each aim for all operations under a category or all operations under *any* category (see later for special considerations). Appropriate weightings have already been included in indicators; however, adjustment for frequency of an operation, f, and case-mix factor, w, for that operation are still necessary to include a fair representation of the true level of quality and performance along the IOM dimensions. Therefore, a category metric (CM) for IOM aim a that includes indicators for aim a for all operations under the category can be calculated as in **Equation 6-3**.

$$CM_a = \frac{\sum_{i=1}^{n} f_i \cdot w_i \cdot I_{a,i}}{\sum_{i=1}^{n} f_i \cdot w_i}$$

Equation 6-3. Category metric (CM) for IOM aim a for a given category of operation.

A metric for each IOM aim for *any* operation category can be calculated from category metrics using a special factor CW that represents the category weight.

CW reflects the relative size and importance of the categories of operation. Therefore, a metric for IOM aim a is calculated as in **Equation 6-4**.

$$M_a = \frac{\sum_{i=1}^{n} CW_i \cdot CM_{a,i}}{\sum_{i=1}^{n} CW_i}$$

Equation 6-4. Metric (M_a) for IOM aim a representing all categories of operations.

Finally, the top metric is an aggregate of all metrics across all dimensions, including a priority factor, U, for each of the IOM aims. This priority factor is important because an organization may give priority to some dimension (IOM aims) (e.g., safety) and may wish this priority reflected in its top quality metric. This metric can be calculated as in **Equation 6-5**.

$$Top\ Metric = \frac{\sum_{i=1}^{6} U_i \cdot M_i}{\sum_{i=1}^{6} U_i}$$

Equation 6-5. Top metric calculation.

As with indicators, metrics for all five domains of access, structure, process, outcome, and patient experience (for a given operation category or for all operations) may also be calculated from the corresponding indicators (**Equations 6-6 and 6-7**). These metrics will provide performance information along those domains to the managers within the organizations; however, they will have little value to the consumers outside the organization. Such metrics may be useful in the planning process and in problem solving.

$$CM_d = \frac{\sum_{i=1}^{n} f_i \cdot w_i \cdot I_{d,i}}{\sum_{i=1}^{n} f_i \cdot w_i}$$

Equation 6-6. Category metric for dimension d for a given operation category.

$$M_d = \frac{\sum_{i=1}^{n} CW_i \cdot CM_{d,i}}{\sum_{i=1}^{n} CW_i}$$

Equation 6-7. Metric for dimension d representing all categories of operations.

Requirements for Implementing the Framework

A property of all of the formulas presented here is that they will have the same upper and lower boundaries of the scoring scheme. Therefore, the metrics, indicators, and measures will have a similar range.

Given this mathematical description and related calculations, it is evident that quantifying the quality of care in an institution is a difficult task from the standpoints of data requirements and calculations. It requires dedicated staff and infrastructure. It is a task not to be underestimated.

Finally, this complex setup is designed to address all contingencies for multiple outcomes and multiple measures. It may be that the number of outcomes of interest may be small. If the measures are not related to all outcomes, the math could quickly decrease in complexity. However, it is important to have a framework in place so new measures can be readily introduced into the system. Organizations could start implementing such a framework by starting with single operation outcomes that are of national, regional, or strategic interest and building a data stream that provides quality information. This information can be used to provide proprietary, private, or public performance reports and also corrective action during strategy development and implementation. It provides conformity across various domains and dimensions and across organizational operations.

THE APPROPRIATE LEVEL OF QUALITY

The Joint Commission has been in existence for many years. TJC sets standards for healthcare organizations and issues accreditation. TJC approval might have been the stamp of quality in the past, but it is no longer sufficient for a competitive healthcare market. TJC's main focus is on the quality and delivery of clinical care, whereas the broader definition of quality entails factors such as efficiency, equity, and patient centeredness.[13]

In today's competitive healthcare market, quality is one of the bases for competing and therefore an essential aspect of organizational strategy. The importance of quality as a strategic and operational management lever continues to grow as the organization gains a better understanding of its meaning, measurement, and improvement. Going back to Kano's model of quality described previously in this text, quality of medical care is a basic requirement; it is the one that *must* exist. Patients assume that it exists. Lack of it will drive consumers away, either through regulatory action or word of mouth from other patients. The provision of efficient and high-value care is a performance requirement.

Improvement of service quality comes as an excitement requirement.[14] Consumers do not expect it, but its existence will improve their satisfaction. Examples of service requirement in a hospital are food services, timely transportation to different areas of the hospital, and accommodations for family. These (hotel) services and related service "quality" implications are not the focus of this text.

In addition to provision of clinical quality, for a healthcare organization to survive it must also be attentive to service delivery, financial viability, and community value.[15]

Thus far, it is obvious that improvement of quality requires metrics and measurements. But metrics and measurements are not the only required components for quality improvement. Operating with high quality requires cultural changes in the organization. Quality of care is affected by variability in the system where the two major sources of variability are:[16]

1. *External variability*: These are differences that cannot be controlled by an operator. Case-mix is the external variable factor of health care.
2. *Internal variability*: These are differences that can be controlled by an operator. Providing a patient with a prescription for aspirin at the time of discharge will not guarantee that the patient will fill the prescription or will take the medication.

In general, health care, including medical care, has substantial internal and external variability. Many of the operations in health care are operator dependent and vary from one operator to another. This is why having checkpoints and mechanisms to capture errors are important in creating a high quality environment.

Tiers of Quality

With the measurement of quality comes the inevitable consequence of having different levels or tiers of quality. Although this may initially seem acceptable as long as the lowest class or tier still meets the minimum standards or expectations, in fact it may create a problem. However, this is not a new problem.

If, for a particular procedure or treatment, there are multiple outcome tiers and therefore quality levels, where the higher tiers represent better outcomes, should this automatically reset the outcome standards and expectations for that particular treatment or procedure? If yes, this would make the lower tiers substandard. Even now, there exist reporting systems that provide information about outcomes for a number of diseases and procedures at different medical centers. Clearly, some will be below the "national average." This effect may even persist after adjusting for input variability through case-mix adjustments. Performing at or above the national average is a reasonable expectation; however, the clear dilemma is that as lower tiers move toward the national average, the average moves away from them.

A reasonable amount of variation can be tolerated. The key is how to define the acceptable range of variation around the national average.

REFERENCES

1. Reeves GR, Wang TY, Reid KJ, et al. Dissociation between hospital performance of the smoking cessation counseling quality metric and cessation outcomes after myocardial infarction. *Arch Intern Med.* 2008;168(19):2111–2117.
2. Davenport DL, Holsapple CW, Conigliaro J. Assessing surgical quality using administrative and clinical data sets: a direct comparison of the University HealthSystem Consortium Clinical Database and the National Surgical Quality Improvement Program data set. *Am J Med Qual.* 2009;24(5):395–402.
3. McDonald KM, Romano PS, Geppert J, et al. Measures of patient safety based on hospital administrative data—the patient safety indicators. http://www.ncbi.nlm.nih .gov/entrez/query.fcgi?cmd=Retrieve&db=PubMed&dopt=Citation&list_uids =20734521. August 2002.
4. Lohr KN. *Medicare: A Strategy for Quality Assurance.* Vol. 1. Washington, DC: Institute of Medicine; 1990.
5. Committee on Quality of Health Care in America. *Crossing the Quality Chasm: A New Health System for the 21st Century.* Washington, DC: Institute of Medicine; 2001.
6. Child health care quality toolbox: understanding quality measurement. Agency for Healthcare Research and Quality website. http://www.ahrq.gov/chtoolbx/understn .htm#whata. Published 2004. Accessed November 4, 2011.
7. CMS. *Roadmap for Quality Measurement in the Traditional Medicare Fee-for-Service Program.* Baltimore, MD: Centers for Medicare & Medicaid Services; 2009.
8. Freeman T. Using performance indicators to improve health care quality in the public sector: a review of the literature. *Health Serv Manage Res.* 2002;15(2):126–137.
9. Center for Health Policy Studies, Harvard School of Public Health, Center for Quality of Care Research, Education. *Understanding and Choosing Clinical Performance Measures for Quality Improvement: Development of Typology: Final Report.* Rockville, MD: Agency for Healthcare Research and Quality; 2007.
10. Lawthers AW, Palmer H, Seltzer J, Nash DB. In search of a few good performance measures. In: *Models for Measuring Quality in Managed Care: Analysis and Impact.* New York, NY: Faulkner & Gray's Healthcare Information Center; 1997:121–150.
11. Domain framework and inclusion criteria. Agency for Healthcare Research and Quality website. http://www.qualitymeasures.ahrq.gov/about/domain-definitions .aspx. Published 2011. Accessed November 5, 2011.
12. Hurtado MP, Institute of Medicine. Committee on Quality of Health Care in America. *Envisioning the National Health Care Quality Report.* Washington, DC: National Academy Press; 2001.

13. Luttman RJ. "Next generation quality": beyond compliance. *Inside Case Management.* 2000;6(10):4–6.

14. Sauerwein EBF, Matzler K, Hinterhuber H. The Kano model: how to delight your customers. *International Working Seminar on Production Economics.* 1996:313–327.

15. Royer TC. Excellence is a necessity, not a luxury. *Front Health Serv Manage.* 2007;23(4):29–32; discussion 43-25.

16. Chao S. *Advancing Quality Improvement Research: Challenges and Opportunities. Workshop Summary.* Washington, DC: National Academy of Sciences; 2007.

CHAPTER 7

Understanding Quality and Performance

INTRODUCTION

From a managerial perspective, organizational success should be defined by the achievement of the organization's performance objectives. Once the organization has defined its view of success in these terms, it needs a plan to achieve the objectives. Clarity with respect to the concepts of performance, performance measurement, and strategy are essential to the effective leadership and management of any organization. With that in mind, it seems appropriate to start by building a foundation on which to develop an understanding of these concepts.

GOALS AND OBJECTIVES

After reading this chapter, the reader should be able to:

1. Define strategy, organizational performance, finance, and quality and their interactions.
2. Discuss accountability within a healthcare organization.
3. Discuss the significance of values, mission, and vision statements for a healthcare organization.
4. Discuss internal factors within and external factors outside the organization that impact quality of care.
5. Define and discuss value in health care.

6. Discuss the strategic decision-making process on the basis of financial metrics.

7. Discuss the strategic decision-making process on the basis of financial and quality metrics and describe a quality equivalent for return on investment (ROI).

PERFORMANCE, STRATEGY, FINANCE, AND QUALITY

Organizational performance, as derived from the mission of the organization, includes both financial and quality considerations—the "two bottom lines" described previously in this text. In the short term, these two components of organizational performance are contained in the general domain of operating performance as reflected in the organizational budgets, whereas longer-term financial and quality measures are bundled under the umbrella of strategic performance, which is expected to result from the successful execution of the organization's strategic plan (**Figure 7-1**).

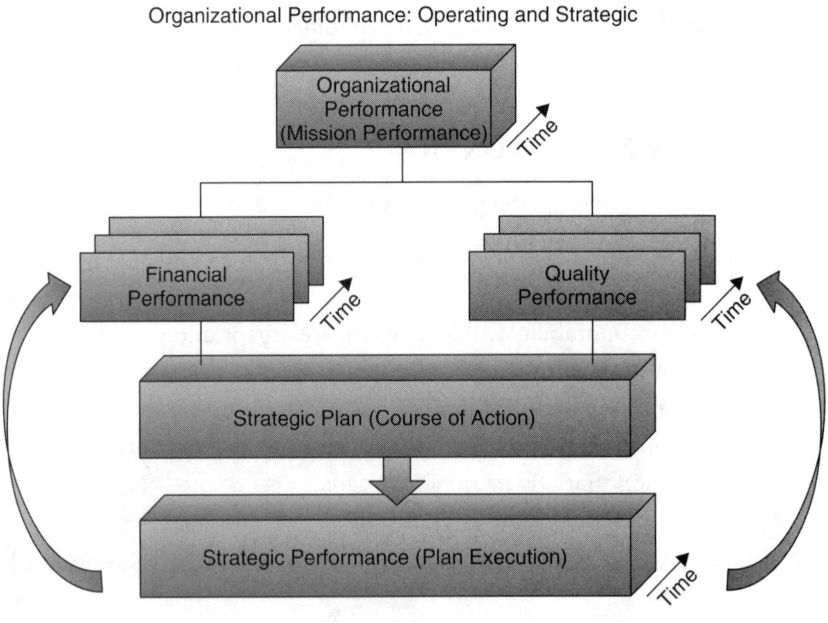

Organizational Performance: Operating and Strategic

FIGURE 7-1. The main components of performance.

Clearly, long-term or strategic performance is represented by an accumulation of a succession of short-term performances. This is true in the case of financial performance and certainly should be the case for quality performance. What should be added to this notion of performance is that to ensure sustainability of financial performance and quality performance over the long term, key initiatives and investments must be undertaken. These key initiatives and investments are the basic elements of strategy and its successful implementation (i.e., the successful execution of strategy is what will ensure long-term, strategic performance). Although in large part the success of a strategy is often measured in financial terms, as goals and targets are usually either set in those terms or are readily translated to financial terms, for many years there has been an awareness of the importance of other indicators of performance such as quality.[1] Given the necessity of financial health, quality has often taken a back seat to finance in the definition and measurement of organizational performance.

Quality as a performance measure is in many ways still in its infancy in the healthcare industry, and perhaps the biggest challenge to its successful integration into this industry is in recognizing its relationship to financial performance. This is similar to the challenges in recognizing and understanding the relationship between strategy and finance, where any new strategy must meet the financial seal of approval before executives can set out on implementation of the strategy. The same principles and conceptual connections apply here, with perhaps one caveat: aside from mounting regulatory pressure in its favor, quality is an increasingly important strategic weapon against the competition.[2]

In traditional strategic planning, the process includes strategic and operational feasibility determination followed by confirmation of financial feasibility before concluding whether the strategic initiative could or should be adopted. Strategic performance, in turn, is assessed in financial terms, and in fact the "value" of a strategy is often described in terms of the financial returns that the strategy produces.

One might argue that any number of quality initiatives could be evaluated through the same process and be adopted or rejected. Furthermore, quality performance could ultimately be assessed in financial terms once the initiative is implemented and course corrections can be executed as needed depending on the level of performance being achieved relative to expectations. It must be recognized that the way in which quality affects financial performance can be quite variable—ranging from provision of efficiencies in the organization's cost structure to improved market position through the delivery of a superior competitive product or service. At the same time, enhanced product or service

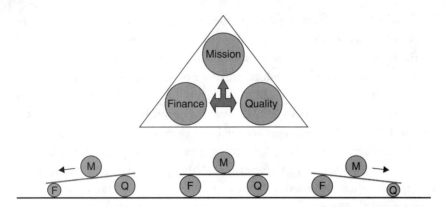

FIGURE 7-2. A balance between finance and quality is required for the success of an organization's mission. M: Mission; F: Finance; Q: Quality.

quality may be more costly, and in that case the offset should be improved market position.

The point of contention here is that quality of care delivered in a healthcare organization is an integral part of the organization; it is in many ways the most important distinguishing attribute of the organization. Therefore, quality of care provided should have at least equal importance to volume measures such as the number of surgeries performed or the number of patient discharges. For this reason, performance along the quality axis must be addressed with the same zeal as that for performance along the finance axis.

If such a balanced view is adopted in the organization, the quality impact of any initiative should be evaluated during strategic and operational feasibility studies, and the final decision should be based on a comprehensive and balanced view of feasibility, not just on financial feasibility.

Assuming such a position, it would naturally follow that it is in fact the interactions between quality and finance (and their corresponding levels of performance) that will provide evidence of the organization's success in fulfilling its mission and accomplishing its strategic goals. Any imbalance that puts too much emphasis on finance or quality at the expense of the other will compromise long-term strategic success and overall mission fulfillment (**Figure 7-2**).

VALUE IN HEALTH CARE

Quality alone is rarely the driving force behind a consumer's choice. Instead, most consumers use a derivative of quality as the basis of their selection of the product or service they will purchase. This derivative is value. A brief discussion of value in health care is central to understanding some of the unique dynamics of consumer–provider interactions in the healthcare system.

Most people when shopping for a product or good look for more than one feature; when buying a computer, it is not just the CPU speed or RAM capacity. At the same time, again for most people, price is also a factor. When looking at all of these considerations, the consumer looks for *value* in comparing features to price—the more features for the same price or the same features at a lower price both suggest higher value to the consumer. Unless one is so wealthy that price is immaterial, value is at the core of our decision making in the purchase and consumption of goods and services.

Why is it, then, that such a basic and commonsense principle is so scarce in health care? Is it possible that it is the unintended result of the way the healthcare system operates?

For most healthcare consumers, and this is perhaps unique to the healthcare industry, the concept of value does not apply. Why? In large part it is because they do not pay directly for health services (except for the out-of-pocket component, which is 22% of total expenditure for privately insured individuals[3]) and frequently are unaware of the charges and reimbursement for the care they receive. As odd as it sounds, most consumers of health services, including physicians, are not aware of the prices of or payment for services, with the possible exception of the above-mentioned out-of-pocket expenses: co-pay, deductible, and co-insurance. Consumers either have some form of private or public healthcare coverage or have no coverage. In either case, they frequently show little sensitivity to price. As a result, important questions such as, "Do I need this test?" or "Is there a less expensive and similarly effective alternative?" seldom get asked. Moreover, they also do not have a full understanding and appreciation of the quality of the health service they are consuming.

For the most part, value can be defined as shown in **Equation 7-1**.

$$\text{Value} \propto \frac{\text{Quality(Benefits)}}{\text{Price}}$$

Equation 7-1. The basic relationship that describes value.

When maximizing value, most shoppers look at this ratio, and this is one of the forces in the free market economy that affects the market share and success or failure of competing organizations. Unfortunately, because payers and consumers are often not the same entity in health care, and because most consumers are unable to discern quality differences, this ratio is not as reflective of consumption behavior as it might be in other industries.

Payers *can* use this equation to contract with providers that provide greater value by reducing price and increasing quality or by increasing quality at a faster rate than that of increase in price. However, which approach is chosen is not determined by the consumer, and in fact the consumer may disagree with the chosen approach.

Another important parameter in the analysis of value in health care is consumers' lack of medical knowledge, resulting in their dependence on physician agents, which is commonly referred to as *asymmetry of information.*[4] This is known to result in overuse (supplier- or, in this case, provider-induced demand) of the resources and reduction in value, unbeknownst to the consumer.[5]

It has been suggested that a better understanding by providers and payers of the relationship between costs and outcomes (i.e., value) may hold the key to controlling the rising costs of the U.S. healthcare system. Indeed, the inability to measure value using the proper costs and proper outcomes is identified as the main reason costs cannot be controlled.[6]

Value is a concept related to cost effectiveness of care. Comparative effectiveness is also an approach to integrate value into the healthcare model. Both of these methods are at the level of policy makers, and perhaps this lack of understanding or involvement of consumers and providers with these concepts is the reason for this issue to be a political minefield.[7-9]

INTERNAL AND EXTERNAL INFLUENCES ON QUALITY

The organization's quality performance is influenced by many factors, some internal to the organization and some external. **Figure 7-3** illustrates some of the more influential factors. An understanding of these factors can contribute significantly to the development and execution of the organization's strategy, as will be seen later in this text. This understanding also can help with the identification of the organization's strengths, weaknesses, opportunities, and threats (SWOT).

Internal Influences

Internal influences are components or characteristics of the organization itself and find meaning only within the context of the organization. They can be considered as strengths or weakness for the organization and can result in creation of opportunities or threats for the organization. Modification of these components or characteristics can be part of an organization's strategy and can result in a change in quality performance.

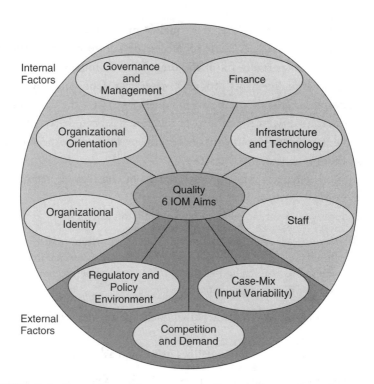

FIGURE 7-3. A number of factors can influence the quality of care delivered in a hospital; some are listed in the illustration.

Organizational Identity

What is the basis for judging the level of performance on a metric in an organization? In other words, what is the expectation for that metric in the context of the organization? This leads to a different question: What is the context or overall purpose of the organization?

This purpose, the rationale for the organization's existence, should be captured in its mission statement.[10,11] Most organizations have statements of values, mission, and vision upon which they build a supporting long-term strategy. These statements can be very helpful in guiding the development of strategy.[12] At the same time, the foundational statements also provide the basis for assessment of organizational performance. It is expected that metrics used by the organization actually provide, directly or indirectly, a means for measuring the organization's fulfillment of mission and therefore a basis for mission accountability. If the metrics do not flow from mission, their usefulness and justification are open to question.

It stands to reason, therefore, that quality must be a *mission* focus for it to be relevant to the assessment of success or failure of a strategic plan that aims to at least partially fulfill the organization's mission by delivering a desired level of quality in its products or services. Consequently, whereas mission incorporates the desire to provide quality services, the determination of whether that quality, in the context of mission, has been delivered is based on achieving the quality targets contained in the performance expectations for the organization.

The mission statements of four organizations of considerable reputation in health care are listed below.

Massachusetts General Hospital declares its mission as[13]:

> Guided by the needs of our patients and their families, we aim to deliver the very best health care in a safe, compassionate environment; to advance that care through innovative research and education; and, to improve the health and well-being of the diverse communities we serve.

One can infer from the above statement that quality of care delivered is of concern to the organization.

M. D. Anderson Cancer Center defines its mission as[14]:

> The mission of The University of Texas M. D. Anderson Cancer Center is to eliminate cancer in Texas, the nation, and the world through outstanding programs that integrate patient care, research and prevention, and through education for undergraduate and graduate students, trainees, professionals, employees and the public.

There is no direct reference to quality in this statement. M. D. Anderson is one of the best cancer centers in the nation, and yet quality is not directly addressed in its mission statement. Of course, with some imagination, one can detect an indirect reference to quality in the above statement; perfection, as in *eliminating cancer*, has a hint of quality in it.

Cleveland Clinic Foundation defines its mission as[15]:

> The mission of Cleveland Clinic is to provide better care of the sick, investigation into their problems, and further education of those who serve.

Quality is not directly referenced in this statement.

Mayo Clinic Foundation defines its mission as[16]:

> To inspire hope and contribute to health and well-being by providing the best care to every patient through integrated clinical practice, education and research.

Quality is directly referenced here as the "best care."

As seen in these mission statements, if quality is not explicitly stated, it does not necessarily translate to lower quality or lack of quality in that organization. However, it does seem reasonable and consistent with best practices to include quality as a core value or part of the mission statement if it indeed is something of which the organization is mindful. At the same time, a reference to quality in the mission statement does not translate to higher quality in the delivery of health services by those organizations—particularly if they do not have a mechanism for "mission accountability."

If quality is incorporated into the mission statement, it will at least provide an explicit basis for inclusion in the organization's strategic planning and positioning and will guide the staff in their daily operations, eventually resulting in higher-quality delivery of care. This in turn may afford the organization a competitive edge. In fact, as suggested earlier, quality may be considered a *strategic weapon*[1] and may even be considered *as* integral to strategy.[17]

The importance of the mission statement in the life of an organization has been discussed for many years. Yet, surprising as it may sound, healthcare organizations appear far behind other industries in using the mission statement to give meaning to their existence. This is not limited to stating their position on quality; it also applies to other concepts such as finance, cost, and access.[18]

Governance and Management

From an organizational perspective, management is delegated the responsibility for the operational and financial functions, and their activities are overseen by a board of directors. The board of directors holds the executive team accountable for compliance with the organization's values and mission while ensuring the organization's path toward its vision by achievement of the performance targets approved by the board (**Figure 7-4**). The one area of shared responsibility, and some contention, is that of strategy development, which links the governance domain with that of management. Embedded in this shared responsibility is the consideration of quality for the organization. For the remainder of this chapter, references to a *board* refer to a board of directors with fiduciary responsibilities, unless specifically stated otherwise.

Quality of care and the role of a board of directors in quality improvement have been the subject of in-depth research. This chapter will focus on some of the more important issues related to the board's role and strategies for its success in quality improvement.

Since publication of the Institute of Medicine (IOM) report *To Err Is Human*,[19] quality of hospital care has come into the national spotlight.

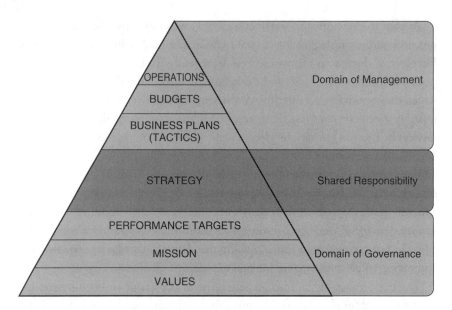

FIGURE 7-4. Strategy is a shared responsibility between the board and the management of an organization. Oversight of management's compliance with the organization's mission and values is the duty of the board. The identity of an organization can best be thought of in two layers: values upon which the organization is built will serve as the motivation for its mission and purpose; mission will specify the organizational purpose and "journey." Vision will articulate the "destination" for the journey on which the organization is embarked. Performance is based on this foundation and should be the basis for progress toward the destination.

Clearly, boards have a fiduciary responsibility for what happens in their organizations and as a result are legally liable for the appropriate discharge of their duties. As such, quality of care is one such duty, and boards are actually liable for the quality of care delivered in their organizations.[20–23] Additionally, a board in a general sense has authority over the management team and can remove or appoint the CEO of the organization. This is a significant lever that a board has in its hands, and a board can use it to steer the organization and affect the direction of quality improvement.[21]

What are the economic and financial costs associated with the pursuit of quality? Is quality expensive? To achieve a higher level of quality, new mechanisms must be put in place; this may require additional staffing, equipment, audits, and so forth. This all costs money. As it turns out, lack of quality may be even more expensive, and there may be, over time or immediately, a net positive economic effect after a higher level of quality is achieved.[24] This business case for quality should place it at the top of a board's agenda.

There are other persuasive arguments for making quality a board priority. National trends demand higher quality of care, and boards should recognize and respond to them in order to ensure the long-term viability of the organization. This suggests not only that the organization's board has a critical role to play in the determination of the organization's quality standards but also that quality should be a key item on the board's agenda.[25–27]

The failure of boards in promoting a quality agenda is multidimensional. It has to do with several different internal and external factors that come to play in the scope of organizational governance. The structure between hospital boards and the medical staff has been blamed for not permitting the boards to monitor the quality for which they are legally responsible.[20] It has been suggested that boards of trustees are legally and ethically responsible for the quality of patient care; however, they do not have the structure and function to know or improve the quality of care. It is imperative to examine and determine whether the current structure facilitates the solution or accentuates the problem.[20]

Still, there is more to this problem. In comparison with the automotive industry, some of the barriers to successful quality improvement in health care include inadequate organizational structure, lack of quality measures, quality improvement indicators focused on nonclinical areas, lack of information, and lack of financial incentives for physicians.[28,29] Lack of external auditing is also a problem.[23] The following is a more comprehensive list of the types of barriers to success that may be encountered by boards when attempting to promote a quality agenda[21]:

1. Barriers related to board members, including lack of understanding of quality on the part of members and the resulting lack of confidence and moral authority to speak on matters of quality.
2. Barriers related to the information available to the board.
3. Barriers related to interactions of the board with the medical staff on matters such as physician competence.
4. Barriers related to lack of priority for quality on the part of the board resulting in lack of investment and delegation to quality committees.

Any board that has built up the will to tackle the enormous challenge of quality improvement should systematically deal with this list and address these barriers before it can successfully pursue a quality agenda.

There have been calls for boards to lead in hospital quality improvement.[21,30] Boards can certainly set the agenda,[31] but this does not necessarily result in successful execution of the agenda.

Boards can be classified as either philanthropic (advisory) or corporate (fiduciary) based on size, perspectives, compensation, management participation and accountability, and strategic activities.[32] To these we can add physician representation, community and constituency representation, and number of committees.[33] Evidence shows that nonprofit hospitals that have corporate-model boards are likely to be more efficient and have more admissions and a larger share of the market,[34,35] yet the specific issue of quality of care and its relationship to the nature of the board was not studied.[34] The organizational infrastructure, however, seems to be related to scope and intensity of the hospital's quality improvement efforts.[36]

There are more general steps that a board can take to address the problems we discussed and increase the chances of success with respect to quality improvement. In a study, executives at 413 hospitals in a number of states were surveyed about their practices. Quality performance data for the 413 hospitals as determined by the CareScience Quality Index was used to evaluate the effect of those practices. Factors associated with better quality included spending greater than 25% of board time on quality, using a formal tool such as a dashboard, compensating senior management for quality, and increasing engagement with the medical staff.[37] A higher percentage of voting medical staff on a board (30.3% vs. 20.8%) was found to be an important difference between a group of high-performing hospitals and a group of average hospitals.[38] Educating the board on quality initiatives appears to be another important factor in preparation for success.[39]

The following is a list of initiatives to counter the list of barriers presented earlier[21]:

1. Educate members on quality and assume a proactive position on quality.
2. Establish quality standards and benchmarks; create a clear and accountable chain of command for quality.
3. Engage the medical staff, establish guidelines, and expect accountability.
4. Give a high priority to quality through strategic planning and action.

Although executive accountability for quality can be considered part of board activism, it is recommended by the Institute for Healthcare Improvement.[30]

In order for boards to do their jobs, as discussed earlier, they need information, mostly in the form of reports, performance measures, and even a performance dashboard. A more detailed discussion of this subject will be presented later on in this text.

A thorough bibliography on the subject of healthcare governance was published in 2007 and is a good resource for further reading.[28]

Organizational Orientation

Generally, organizations, including healthcare organizations, can be divided into three distinct groups: governmental, nonprofit, and for-profit. This grouping is referred to here as the organization's orientation. The role and impact of this orientation on the quality of care delivered has been a topic of discussion and at times controversy. Some of the highlights of organizational orientation, specifically for-profit and nonprofit, are presented in the following paragraphs. Governmental organizations (public) are slightly different and are not discussed here. They include the Veterans Health Administration (VHA) system and state-, county-, and city-owned hospitals, among others.

One would imagine that there should be no difference in quality between the two nongovernmental (private) orientations. Perhaps for-profit organizations would be more expensive, maybe even more exclusive of nonpaying patients, but in that case the quality should be better or on a par with that of nonprofit organizations.

What about shareholder expectations and profits? It is not inconceivable that management in a for-profit organization may be under pressure to maximize profits, and this *may* in turn influence the quality of care delivered. As Kenneth J. Arrow suggested in 1963, it could be that nonprofit organizations represent higher quality of care and that the very word *profit* is a signal that denies trust.[40] It may be that in the context of for-profit organizations, quality is but a means to financial success. Nonprofit organizations, in contrast, may see financial performance as a means to invest in and improve quality. Despite the differences in orientation, today nonprofit and for-profit organizations share more similarities than differences in both the financial and quality dimensions as a result of competitive and regulatory pressures.

In one study, quality of care was measured in terms of survival, changes in functional and cognitive status, and living arrangements; the results of this study did not show a difference between nonprofit and for-profit hospitals caring for Medicare patients, although payments were found to be higher to for-profit hospitals.[41]

Additionally, it has been suggested that the government orientation of hospitals, as well as whether they are nonprofit or for-profit, may have an impact on the services they provide and also on their patient mix; however, the effect on quality of care is not examined in detail.[42] Another study has found that the incidence of adverse outcomes is 3% to 4% higher in government and for-profit hospitals compared with that in nonprofit hospitals.[43] The same study also shows that conversion from nonprofit to for-profit—which could happen for various reasons and through different mechanisms—is associated with a 7% to 9% increase in adverse outcomes.[43]

In a meta-analysis of 15 observational studies involving more than 26,000 hospitals and 38 million patients, the mortality rate of patients in private for-profit hospitals was found to be higher than that of patients in private nonprofit hospitals.[44] Despite these findings, it appears that once adjustments are made for patient-mix, factors other than for-profit status per se may be the main determinants of quality of care (outcomes) in hospitals.[45]

The impact of organizational orientation on quality may be more prominent in contexts other than hospitals. Data from other studies looking at the differences in quality and/or mortality in dialysis centers show a higher mortality associated with for-profit status.[46] There is a suggestion in the literature that for-profit nursing homes may have more deficiencies, although other studies have shown little or no difference.[47,48]

One could expand this question to payers as well. Investor-owned Health Maintenance Organizations (HMOs) were shown to have lower quality of care compared with that of nonprofit HMOs.[49] There is also further evidence that links financial pressure to poor quality of care.[50,51]

Finance

A review and synthesis of the literature in 2006 examined the empirical evidence of the association between quality and finance in healthcare organizations using the original Donabedian framework of structure, process, and outcome. Some of the findings are discussed here with citation of the original sources.[52]

Multiple studies have identified a link between hospitals' expenses and outcomes. These expenses were divided between patient care and administration. Although most studies found that a higher relative expenditure on patient care may be associated with better outcomes,[53–55] the opposite was true with respect to administrative expenditures at the level of the provider institution or health plan.[56,57] Higher financial margin also seems to be associated with higher quality perhaps because the organization has more latitude to support quality efforts compared with the competition.[55,58]

The effect of financial performance on structure and quality is not as well studied as the relationship to outcomes, but there seems to be an association. In one study, better financial support allowed healthcare organizations to invest in structural quality that resulted in higher accreditation status by The Joint Commission.[59]

Similarly, there seems to be a positive association between higher medical spending, profitability, and fiscal margins and process measures of quality. Availability of financial resources resulted in increased use of preventive and wellness measures and decreased lengths of stay.[52,59,60]

Staff

The dynamics of physician and nurse staffing and quality of care within a healthcare organization is complex. Earlier, the role of interaction between governance, management, and medical staff in quality of care was discussed. But the impact of the medical staff on quality of care does not end there. Physicians and nurses deliver the care on a daily basis, and as a result several factors such as job satisfaction, workload, and awareness directly influence the quality of care.

A meta-analysis of studies of nurse staffing and quality of care showed that there is an association between higher registered nurse (RN) staffing and lower risk of hospital-related mortality and adverse patient events.[61] More hours of nursing care or a higher proportion of care provided by RNs was also found to be associated with better outcomes.[62] However, there is no "fixed" ratio of nurses to patients that provides optimal quality of care.[63] A literature review of the association between patient outcomes and nurse staffing in the critical care setting also reports similar findings.[64]

Similar issues exist in physician staffing. For instance, studies have shown that outcomes are better in the closed ICU models where patients are primarily managed by critical care specialists compared with those of open ICU models with as-needed consultations from the critical care specialists.[65,66] A systematic review of the effect of hospitalist physicians on the quality of care and outcomes also suggests that hospitalist staffing may improve efficiency and decrease length of stay while providing quality of care comparable to that of the traditional staffing models.[67]

Infrastructure and Technology

Infrastructure and technology is a broad category and constitutes the enabling capabilities that allow healthcare organizations to deliver care. But perhaps the component of infrastructure technology with the most extensive reach within the organization is the technology used to store and share information; that is, electronic health records (EHRs). EHRs have become an important part of the modern healthcare system in the United States. In February 2009, President Obama signed the American Recovery and Reinvestment Act of 2009. Title XIII of this legislation is the Health Information Technology for Economic and Clinical Health Act (HITECH act), which allocates approximately $20 billion to EHR adoption in the United States.[68] It is hoped that this investment will increase the adoption of EHRs by healthcare organizations and physicians.

EHRs can play a role in healthcare quality in two important ways. First, EHRs will store data that can be used for measurement of quality in ways that could not be accomplished with paper charts. As will be discussed later in this text, measures of quality can be used in real time to monitor quality status, and this is possible if there is appropriate information technology infrastructure. It is noteworthy that to measure quality properly, one must move away from administrative measures that may reflect quality by proxy such as billing data. The importance of quality in the delivery of care suggests that it is time quality had measures of its own rather than simply relying on billing and claims data.

Second, EHRs could offer significant tools to clinicians for processing of patient data and could offer relevant guidelines and best practices information to clinicians. In theory, EHRs should contribute to quality improvement in a healthcare organization by reducing error, providing decision support capability, and promoting evidence-based practices. However, in empirical studies of the role of EHRs in healthcare quality, a positive contribution has not been verified.[69–71] Furthermore, successful implementation of decision support systems in an EHR will not necessarily mean they will be used.[72,73] There are even reports of increased adverse outcomes after implementation of EHRs.[74]

Realistically, one must acknowledge that EHRs are here to stay. Even though they have not yet delivered on the quality of care aspect of their justification for existence, the healthcare system cannot revert to paper charts. It may be that with a change in culture as well as new and improved software design, some of these promises will be fulfilled. To that end, the $20 billion investment signed into law by President Obama may just be the push needed to overcome this hurdle.

External Influences

External influences are factors that are external to an organization. They can be considered as opportunities or threats to the organization and may point out strengths or weaknesses within the organization. Modification of these factors is typically (unless in extreme situations) beyond the capabilities of an organization, but they do have an impact on the organization's quality performance.

Regulatory and Policy Environment

This covers a broad array of topics, some of which were discussed in some detail previously in this text. However, for the purposes of this discussion, a major policy tool (i.e., incentives) is briefly discussed.

The Centers for Medicare & Medicaid Services (CMS) has been the architect of payment structures in the United States mainly because it is the largest payer in the healthcare system. In new attempts to bring costs under control and increase quality of care delivered, the pay-for-performance (P4P) framework, also known as value-based purchasing (VBP), was introduced to represent positive incentives for improved quality performance.[75] This was followed by the announcement of nonpayment for preventable complications during hospitalization.[76]

Despite the appeal of the idea of linking financial incentives, negative or positive, to quality of care, the empirical evidence has challenged the notion that P4P will result in better outcomes.[77,78] Improvement of performance on the part of providers often translates to more time spent with patients or other forms of investment such as information technology, which may not be recovered through the incentives. This is further complicated by the unintended changes in practice patterns that range from up-coding to denial of surgery for high-risk patients as a result of publicly reported outcomes. In the end, the question seems to be what is the most cost-effective way of implementing VBP and not whether VBP is needed.[79,80]

In its latest iteration of VBP, CMS will reduce hospital reimbursements by 1% and 2% in fiscal years 2013 and 2017. Any savings through reduced reimbursement will be used as incentives for higher-performance hospitals. This translates to an estimated $850 million in redistribution of payments (i.e., bonus payments are capped at the amount saved by reduced payments). This will be expanded to apply to other providers as well.[81,82]

Other relevant aspects of these negative and positive incentives are discussed later in this text. However, it is important to emphasize the fact that if used properly and creatively, these incentives can bring about change in practices and represent a strong link between financial performance and quality improvement.

Competition and Demand

Competition (to provide supply) and demand are two fundamental economic factors that affect market dynamics. They also are essential considerations in decisions to enter or exit a market and in formulation of strategy for large or small healthcare organizations. The association between competition (and demand, which is related but different) and quality has been studied, mostly in the context of managed care with mixed results. A study of the effects of hospital competition and HMO penetration in three states—California, New York, and Wisconsin—on 30-day mortality from acute myocardial infarction, hip fracture, stroke, gastrointestinal bleeding, heart failure, and diabetes mellitus reported lower mortality in California and New York but not in Wisconsin. This effect on outcome (quality) was attributed to competition in the case of California and New York. The report also suggests that HMO penetration in various geographic markets affects outcomes differently. In the case of California, higher HMO penetration was associated with lower mortality, whereas in New York, it was associated with higher mortality.[83] Examination of the effects of competition and HMO penetration in California demonstrated lower 30-day mortality rates in 3 to 5 of the 6 conditions, underlining the fact that such findings may not be generalizable without further investigation.[84]

A systematic review of evidence from the National Health Service of the United Kingdom identifies similar inconsistencies, generally finding that competition is ineffective in improvement of quality. This is perhaps attributable to targeting the wrong quality measure. Two of the studies reviewed found that competition reduced waiting times for myocardial infarction; however, it increased hospital mortality, clearly an inferior outcome representing inferior quality of care. The results of this systematic review, although interesting, may not be generalizable to the U.S. market, and the consumer choice is far more restricted in the U.K. National Health Service than it is in the United States, which affects competition.[85]

In addition to the effect of demand and competition on quality of care, they may also have an effect on prices that in turn affect quality of care. In this complex dynamic, economic theory predicts lower prices and quality as a result of competition—a market condition seen in the United Kingdom. In contrast, where prices are fixed, such as in the United States, economic theory predicts higher quality as a result of competition.[86] Clearly, in an era of policy changes in the U.S. healthcare system, empirical studies should examine the actual role of competition and demand rather than their theoretical effects.

Case-Mix

When patients are hospitalized under a diagnosis-related group (DRG), the treatment options, risks and benefits ratios, average operating cost, and potential outcomes are affected by the secondary DRGs (i.e., comorbidities). This is commonly referred to as case-mix and is used to create a case-mix index (CMI), a weighted index of the volume of discharges, distribution of DRGs, and a weight for intensity of the DRGs. The CMI is used in the Prospective Payment System (PPS) administered by CMS.[87] As expected, outcomes in tertiary healthcare systems are also affected by case-mix necessitating an appropriate statistical adjustment.

How a case-mix adjustment should be done is less clear, and it appears that using the CMI used by CMS for payments may not be the optimal solution.

A study of New York City municipal and voluntary hospitals found that estimates of mortality differences between the two groups are substantially affected by which secondary diagnoses are used in case-mix adjustment.[88] Other factors not included in the CMI also seem to have effects on the outcomes of care. A study of general medicine patients in the setting of a teaching hospital found that the functional status of a patient affects outcomes beyond the physiologic comorbidities and suggested that case-mix adjustment methods may be improved by inclusion of measures of function for patients.[89]

INTEGRATION OF QUALITY AND FINANCE

The discussion to this point has highlighted the fact that quality and finance are equally important and potentially related dimensions of the organization's overall mission performance. Further discussion of the interaction and integration of the two is necessary to better understand this relationship.

The relationship between quality and cost almost seems intuitive. Yet, the connection to the strategic planning process in a healthcare organization has not been adequately made thus far. In manufacturing, in contrast, experts acknowledged this connection as early as 1956. For the first time, the concept of *quality cost*, or lack of quality, emerged and became part of the discussion.[90] Later, other scholars in the field of quality added their own twist to this concept; however, the basic idea has remained the same.[91,92] The cost of quality refers to the cost associated with conformance as well as nonconformance to quality requirements.[92,93] Some have suggested that this cost is the best way to measure quality[93]; a variant of the same concept is cost of poor quality (COPQ).[94]

These efforts, however, were primarily targeted at the manufacturing industries. Manufacturing processes can be monitored for their output variations. Using statistical methods, the significant variations can be distinguished from background noise. As discussed previously in this text, this process is referred to as statistical process control (SPC) and was used successfully by W. Edwards Deming and Walter A. Shewhart during World War II and later in reconstruction of Japan.[95,96] Building on SPC, *process capability* was defined as the ability of a process to produce output within specification limits, and *process capability index* is one of the statistical indicators used to measure process quality.[97] In manufacturing, these specification limits are defined within a spread of six standard deviations between upper and lower boundaries of acceptable process output.[97] Quality cost can be thought of as the cost associated with making a process *capable*.

These concepts, which are at the core of the Six Sigma methodology, are also being tried in the healthcare industry. It is important to note also that the Six Sigma methodology has not been very successful even in the manufacturing industries.[98] It remains to be seen what percentage of healthcare processes lend themselves to Six Sigma methodology considering the fact that healthcare processes are often more complex and have a much larger human element that is harder to control, not only in patients but also in providers. It may be easier to implement SPC or Six Sigma methods in selected areas of health care such as radiation therapy[99] or reduction in length of hospitalization for common conditions.[100]

As it may have become evident by now, these connections between quality and cost, and therefore financial performance, are at the level of individual healthcare processes. Somehow, these considerations, associated with the many processes that require change or improvement, must reach the planning level within the organization. As such, these processes provide part of the link between quality and finance. To appreciate fully the effects of finance on quality and vice versa, a broader approach is required. In the following paragraphs, a general paradigm for such an approach is discussed.

Strategic Decision Making

The choice among different projects or even strategies should be governed by a defined methodology to ensure some consistency in the decision process.

In choosing among different projects, the organization must determine the feasibility of those projects before making the selection. The three components of feasibility are strategic feasibility, operational feasibility, and financial feasibility, which should be considered in that order. When it is determined that a project is consistent with an organization's strategic priorities and the organization has the operational ability to undertake the project, the decision will then depend on financial feasibility. The projects that have successfully met the first two feasibility criteria will be weighed against one another in terms of their financial returns, and the selection will be made.

If a strategy is thought of as a series of coordinated projects, one could see the added complexity of evaluating a strategy, or more accurately a strategic plan. It is best to consider alternate strategic plans in terms of their feasibility in the same way that projects are evaluated.

Financial Decision Metrics

In the financial analysis and feasibility study of a strategic plan, a number of methods can be used to determine the financial returns; however, two methods are more popular than others. These two are the net present value (NPV) method and the internal rate of return (IRR) method. One caveat is that when used to compare mutually exclusive projects, these methods may have conflicting results under certain conditions.[101] Under such conditions, the NPV method is preferred. Alternate strategic plans, given the size of resources they require, may well be mutually exclusive. Therefore, the NPV method should be used in evaluating the financial returns of alternate *strategic plans*. However, there may be a preference for the use of the IRR method for evaluation of *projects*. Therefore, IRR will also be discussed here.

The NPV method relies on discounted cash flow (DCF) technique to determine the net present value of the strategic plan over its life period given the cost of capital or hurdle rate r (**Equation 7-2**).

$$NPV = \sum_{t=0}^{n} \frac{CF_t}{(1+r)^t}$$

Equation 7-2. NPV is net present value; CF_t is cash flow at time index t; and r is the hurdle rate.

If the NPV is a positive number, it will make money for the organization. The strategic plan with the highest NPV should be adopted, *ceteris paribus*.

In contrast, the IRR of a strategy is the discount rate at which the strategy's NPV equals zero (**Equation 7-3**).

$$NPV = \sum_{t=0}^{n} \frac{CF_t}{(1+IRR)^t} = 0$$

Equation 7-3. NPV is net present value; CF_t is cash flow at time index t; and IRR is internal rate of return.

If a strategy has an IRR that exceeds the cost of capital for the organization, or the *hurdle rate*, it will be profitable for the organization and therefore will pass the test of financial feasibility. Assuming that the strategy is operationally feasible, the organization may consider adopting the strategy.

It is important to remember that organizations will have to include adjustments for risk of successful execution of the strategy into their hurdle rate. This is true for both the NPV and IRR methods.

The difference between the IRR and the hurdle rate determines the net return on investment (net ROI) for the project or strategy. A positive net ROI signals the potential for the organization to make money when the strategy is successfully executed (**Equation 7-4**).

$$\text{Net ROI} = \text{IRR} - r_{\text{hurdle}}$$

Equation 7-4. Relationship between internal rate of return (IRR), hurdle rate (r_{hurdle}), and net return on investment (ROI).

Perhaps this intuitive translation of the IRR to net ROI is the reason for its popularity among executives.

The NPV can also be used to calculate an ROI for the strategic plan, although the resulting ROI cannot be used to compare alternate strategic plans. This is because the absolute size of the return is also a consideration. A strategy that uses the full resources of an organization with a smaller ROI may be preferable to a mutually exclusive strategy that has a larger ROI but uses only part of the resources.

Quality Decision Metrics

Similarly, in a quality–finance integrated framework for strategic planning, an ROI for quality could be envisioned. A prerequisite for creating such an index would be having in place a robust, comprehensive, and valid quality monitoring system that is directly tailored to the organization. Such a system could produce quality performance measures, indicators, and metrics for each of the six IOM aims, which can, in turn, be formulated into a single composite metric of the organization's quality standing; this was discussed in more detail earlier in this text. Any change to this metric, as a result of a new strategy, could then be measured with respect to the size of investment that the strategy calls for (i.e., producing a return on investment in terms of quality, or qROI). If necessary, the change in composite quality metric could be adjusted for risks to successful completion of strategy in achieving all of its goals, and therefore a risk-adjusted qROI can be produced.

Financial ROI in conjunction with qROI, or risk-adjusted qROI, would make a stronger and more reasonable determinant of whether the strategy is the correct course of action for the organization. These numbers could also allow for optimization of the planning process, as they can be traced back to their sources—particularly if the source was based on quality improvement. Modification to the sources or plan could allow fine tuning of the execution of the plan.

To illustrate the approach to the evaluation of alternative strategies, consider making a final choice among three strategic initiatives. Assume all three are equally complex requiring similar combinations of resources and have met the operational and financial feasibility tests, and assume that each of these strategies is compatible with the organization's values and mission. Traditionally, the only remaining question about these alternatives would be the NPV or ROI, and the one with the highest NPV or ROI would be the optimal strategy. Using the proposed qROI or risk-adjusted qROI, the organization will have at its disposal another piece of information that can play into which strategy will be chosen. Depending on an organization's priorities, a larger general improvement in qROI (as a percentage improvement in the overall quality metric) may be preferable, and the strategy that provides a lower but reasonable ROI may be selected. It is also possible to have an array of qROIs, or risk-adjusted qROIs, for a number of metrics such as patient safety or timeliness of care and find the optimal strategy according to the organization's priorities.

As might be expected, it must be anticipated that changes in quality will have financial implications and vice versa. Therefore, in evaluating a strategy, such implications should be considered, and an equilibrium point where iterative effects of changes in quality on finance and vice versa have all been accounted for should be envisioned. This will be discussed later in this text.

REFERENCES

1. Eccles RG. The performance measurement manifesto. *Harvard Business Review.* 1991; 69(1):131–137.
2. Garvin DA. Competing on the eight dimensions of quality. *Harvard Business Review.* 1987;65(6):101–109.
3. Trends in health care costs and spending. Kaiser Family Foundation website. http://www.kff.org/insurance/upload/7692_02.pdf. Published March 2009. Accessed May 10, 2009.
4. Folland S, Goodman A, Stano M. Asymmetric information and agency. In: *The Economics of Health and Health Care.* Vol 5. Englewood Cliffs, NJ: Prentice Hall; 2007: 199–214.
5. Folland S, Goodman A, Stano M. The physician's practice. In: *The Economics of Health and Health Care.* Vol 5. Englewood Cliffs, NJ: Prentice Hall; 2007:313–330.
6. Kaplan RS, Porter ME. How to solve the cost crisis in health care. *Harvard Business Review.* 2011;89(9):46–52, 54, 56–61 passim.
7. Avorn J. Debate about funding comparative-effectiveness research. *N Engl J Med.* 2009; 360(19):1927–1929.
8. Garber AM, Tunis SR. Does comparative-effectiveness research threaten personalized medicine? *N Engl J Med.* 2009;360(19):1925–1927.
9. Naik AD, Petersen LA. The neglected purpose of comparative-effectiveness research. *N Engl J Med.* 2009;360(19):1929–1931.
10. McCartney JJ. Values based decision making in healthcare: introduction. *HEC Forum.* 2005;17(1):1–5.
11. Iltis AS. Values based decision making in healthcare: organizational mission and integrity. *HEC Forum.* 2005;17(1):6–17.
12. Mills AE, Spencer EM. Values based decision making in healthcare: a tool for achieving the goals of healthcare. *HEC Forum.* 2005;17(1):18–32.

13. Hospital overview. Massachusetts General Hospital website. http://www.massgeneral.org/about/overview.aspx. Published 2011. Accessed November 6, 2011.

14. Mission and values. MD Anderson Cancer Center website. http://www.mdanderson.org/about-us/strategic-vision/mission-and-values/index.html. Published 2011. Accessed November 6, 2011.

15. Mission, vision and values. Cleveland Clinic website. http://my.clevelandclinic.org/about-cleveland-clinic/overview/who-we-are/mission-vision-values.aspx. Published 2009. Accessed November 6, 2011.

16. Mayo Clinic mission and values. Mayo Clinic website. http://www.mayoclinic.org/about/missionvalues.html. Published 2011. Accessed November 6, 2011.

17. Garvin D. Competing on the eight dimensions of quality. *Harvard Business Review.* 1987.

18. Bolon DS. Comparing mission statement content in for-profit and not-for-profit hospitals: does mission really matter? *Hosp Top.* 2005;83(4):2–9.

19. Kohn LC, J, Donaldson M. *To Err Is Human: Building a Safer Health System.* Washington, DC: National Academy Press; 2000.

20. Marren JP, Feazell GL, Paddock MW. The hospital board at risk and the need to restructure the relationship with the medical staff: bylaws, peer review and related solutions. *Ann Health Law.* 2003;12(2):179–234, table.

21. Gautam KS. A call for board leadership on quality in hospitals. *Qual Manag Health Care.* 2005;14(1):18–30.

22. Gosfield AG, Reinertsen JL. The 100,000 Lives Campaign: crystallizing standards of care for hospitals. *Health Aff (Millwood.).* 2005;24(6):1560–1570.

23. Marren JP. The trustee's responsibility for quality care. *Trustee.* 2004;57(7):26, 28.

24. Feazell GL, Marren JP. The quality-value proposition in health care. *J Health Care Finance.* 2003;30(2):1–29.

25. Bader B. Quality begins in the boardroom. *Mod Healthc.* 2000;30(3):26.

26. Hollingsworth AT, Harper D. Quality: the key issue for the board. *Trustee.* 2001;54(10):38–39.

27. McDonagh KJ. Hospital governing boards: a study of their effectiveness in relation to organizational performance. *J Healthc Manag.* 2006;51(6):377–389.

28. Clough J, Nash DB. Health care governance for quality and safety: the new agenda. *Am J Med Qual.* 2007;22(3):203–213.

29. Coye MJ. No Toyotas in health care: why medical care has not evolved to meet patients' needs. *Health Aff (Millwood.).* 2001;20(6):44–56.

30. 5 Million Lives Campaign. Getting started kit: governance leadership "boards on board" how-to guide. IHI website. http://www.ihi.org/knowledge/Knowledge%20Center%20Assets/Tools%20-%20How-toGuideGovernanceLeadershipGetBoardsonBoards_fc4a672d-d040-4418-867a-947b4d42aba8/HowtoGuideGovernance-BoardsonBoard.aspx. Published 2011. Accessed November 6, 2011.

31. Byrnes JJ. Viewpoint: the board of directors' role in quality improvement. *Healthc Leadersh Manag Rep.* 2001;9(9):10–11.

32. Alexander JA, Ye Y, Lee SY, Weiner BJ. The effects of governing board configuration on profound organizational change in hospitals. *J Health Soc Behav.* 2006;47(3):291–308.

33. Weiner BJ, Alexander JA. Corporate and philanthropic models of hospital governance: a taxonomic evaluation. *Health Serv Res.* 1993;28(3):325–355.

34. Alexander JA, Lee SY. Does governance matter? Board configuration and performance in not-for-profit hospitals. *Milbank Q.* 2006;84(4):733–758.

35. Alexander JA, Lee SY, Wang V, Margolin FS. Changes in the monitoring and oversight practices of not-for-profit hospital governing boards 1989-2005: evidence from three national surveys. *Med Care Res Rev.* 2009;66(2):181–196.

36. Alexander JA, Weiner BJ, Shortell SM, Baker LC, Becker MP. The role of organizational infrastructure in implementation of hospitals' quality improvement. *Hosp Top.* 2006; 84(1):11–20.

37. Vaughn T, Koepke M, Kroch E, Lehrman W, Sinha S, Levey S. Engagement of leadership in quality improvement initiatives: executive quality improvement survey results. *J Patient Saf.* 2006;2(1):2–9.

38. Prybil LD. Size, composition, and culture of high-performing hospital boards. *Am J Med Qual.* 2006;21(4):224–229.

39. Joshi MS, Hines SC. Getting the board on board: engaging hospital boards in quality and patient safety. *Jt Comm J Qual Patient Saf.* 2006;32(4):179–187.

40. Arrow KJ. Uncertainty and the welfare economics of medical care. *American Economic Review.* 1963;53(5):941–973.

41. Sloan FA, Picone GA, Taylor DH, Chou SY. Hospital ownership and cost and quality of care: is there a dime's worth of difference? *J Health Econ.* 2001;20(1):1–21.

42. Horwitz J. Making profits and providing care: comparing nonprofit, for-profit, and government hospitals. Discussion of the value of nonprofit hospital ownership must account for the differences in service offerings among hospital types. *Health Affairs.* 2005;24(3):790–801.

43. Shen Y-C. The effect of hospital ownership choice on patient outcomes after treatment for acute myocardial infarction. *J Health Econ.* 2002;21(5):901–922.

44. Devereaux PJ, Choi PT, Lacchetti C, et al. A systematic review and meta-analysis of studies comparing mortality rates of private for-profit and private not-for-profit hospitals. *CMAJ.* 2002;166(11):1399–1406.

45. McClellan M, Staiger D, Cutler DM. Comparing hospital quality at for-profit and not-for-profit hospitals. In: *The Changing Hospital Industry: Comparing Not-for-Profit and for-Profit Institutions.* Chicago, IL: University of Chicago Press; 2000:93–112.

46. Devereaux PJ, Schunemann HJ, Ravindran N, et al. Comparison of mortality between private for-profit and private not-for-profit hemodialysis centers: a systematic review and meta-analysis. *JAMA.* 2002;288(19):2449–2457.

47. Chesteen S, Helgheim B, Randall T, Wardell D. Comparing quality of care in non-profit and for-profit nursing homes: a process perspective. *Journal of Operations Management.* 2005;23(2):229–242.

48. O'Neill C, Harrington C, Kitchener M, Saliba D. Quality of care in nursing homes: an analysis of relationships among profit, quality, and ownership. *Med Care.* 2003; 41(12):1318–1330.

49. Himmelstein DU, Woolhandler S, Hellander I, Wolfe SM. Quality of care in investor-owned vs not-for-profit HMOs. *JAMA.* 1999;282(2):159–163.

50. Beauvais B, Wells R, Vasey J, Dellifraine JL. Does money really matter? The effects of fiscal margin on quality of care in military treatment facilities. *Hosp Top.* 2007; 85(3):2–15.

51. Shen Y-C. The effect of financial pressure on the quality of care in hospitals. *J Health Econ.* 2003;22(2):243–269.

52. Beauvais B, Wells R. Does money really matter? A review of the literature on the relationships between healthcare organization finances and quality. *Hosp Top*. 2006; 84(2):20–28.

53. Kuhn EM, Hartz AJ, Gottlieb MS, Rimm AA. The relationship of hospital characteristics and the results of peer review in six large states. *Med Care*. 1991;29(10): 1028–1038.

54. Cleverley W, Harvey R. Is there a link between hospital profit and quality? *Healthcare Financial Management*. 1992;46(9):40–45.

55. Burstin HR, Lipsitz SR, Udvarhelyi IS, Brennan TA. The effect of hospital financial characteristics on quality of care. *JAMA*. 1993;270(7):845–849.

56. Himmelstein DU, Woolhandler S. Taking care of business: HMOs that spend more on administration deliver lower-quality care. *Int J Health Serv*. 2002;32(4):657–667.

57. McCormick D, Himmelstein DU, Woolhandler S, Wolfe SM, Bor DH. Relationship between low quality-of-care scores and HMOs' subsequent public disclosure of quality-of-care scores. *JAMA*. 2002;288(12):1484–1490.

58. Encinosa WE, Bernard DM. Hospital finances and patient safety outcomes. *Inquiry*. 2005;42(1):60–72.

59. Langland-Orban B, Gapenski LC, Vogel WB. Differences in characteristics of hospitals with sustained high and sustained low profitability. *Hosp Health Serv Adm*. 1996;41(3):385–399.

60. Born P, Geckler C. HMO quality and financial performance: is there a connection? *J Health Care Finance*. 1998;24(2):65–77.

61. Kane RL, Shamliyan TA, Mueller C, Duval S, Wilt TJ. The association of registered nurse staffing levels and patient outcomes: systematic review and meta-analysis. *Med Care*. 2007;45(12):1195–1204.

62. Needleman J, Buerhaus P, Mattke S, Stewart M, Zelevinsky K. Nurse-staffing levels and the quality of care in hospitals. *N Engl J Med*. 2002;346(22):1715–1722.

63. White KM. Policy spotlight: staffing plans and ratios. *Nurs Manag*. 2006;37(4): 18–22, 24.

64. Penoyer DA. Nurse staffing and patient outcomes in critical care: a concise review. *Crit Care Med*. 2010;38(7):1521–1528; quiz 1529.

65. Pronovost PJ, Angus DC, Dorman T, Robinson KA, Dremsizov TT, Young TL. Physician staffing patterns and clinical outcomes in critically ill patients: a systematic review. *JAMA*. 2002;288(17):2151–2162.

66. Gajic O, Afessa B, Hanson AC, et al. Effect of 24-hour mandatory versus on-demand critical care specialist presence on quality of care and family and provider satisfaction in the intensive care unit of a teaching hospital. *Crit Care Med*. 2008;36(1):36–44.

67. White HL, Glazier RH. Do hospitalist physicians improve the quality of inpatient care delivery? A systematic review of process, efficiency and outcome measures. *BMC Med*. 2011;9:58.

68. American Recovery and Reinvestment Act of 2009. The First Session. ed 2009.

69. Zhou L, Soran CS, Jenter CA, et al. The relationship between electronic health record use and quality of care over time. *J Am Med Inform Assoc*. 2009;16(4):457–464.

70. Keyhani S, Hebert PL, Ross JS, Federman A, Zhu CW, Siu AL. Electronic health record components and the quality of care. *Med Care*. 2008;46(12):1267–1272.

71. Linder JA, Ma J, Bates DW, Middleton B, Stafford RS. Electronic health record use and the quality of ambulatory care in the United States. *Arch Intern Med*. 2007; 167(13):1400–1405.

72. Goldstein MK, Coleman RW, Tu SW, et al. Translating research into practice: organizational issues in implementing automated decision support for hypertension in three medical centers. *J Am Med Inform Assoc.* 2004;11(5):368–376.

73. Schnipper JL, Linder JA, Palchuk MB, et al. "Smart forms" in an electronic medical record: documentation-based clinical decision support to improve disease management. *J Am Med Inform Assoc.* 2008;15(4):513–523.

74. Walker JM, Carayon P, Leveson N, et al. EHR safety: the way forward to safe and effective systems. *J Am Med Inform Assoc.* 2008;15(3):272–277.

75. Committee on Redesigning Health Insurance Performance Measures, Performance Improvement. *Rewarding Provider Performance: Aligning Incentives in Medicare.* Washington, DC: Institute of Medicine; 2006.

76. CMS. Medicare program; changes to the hospital inpatient prospective payment systems and fiscal year 2008 rates. *Fed Reg.* 2007;72(162):47129–48175.

77. Jha AK, Joynt KE, Orav EJ, Epstein AM. The long-term effect of premier pay for performance on patient outcomes. *N Engl J Med.* April 26, 2012;366(17):1606–1615.

78. Fonarow GC, Peterson ED. Heart failure performance measures and outcomes: real or illusory gains. *JAMA.* August 19, 2009;302(7):792–794.

79. Rosenthal MB, Frank RG. What is the empirical basis for paying for quality in health care? *Med Care Res Rev.* 2006;63(2):135–157.

80. Rosenthal MB, Frank RG, Li Z, Epstein AM. Early experience with pay-for-performance: from concept to practice. *JAMA.* 2005;294(14):1788–1793.

81. Ferman JH. Value-based purchasing program here to stay: payments will be based on performance. *Healthc Exec.* 2011;26(3):76, 78.

82. Ferman JH. Value-based purchasing program. Part II. Payments will be based on performance. *Healthc Exec.* 2011;26(4):64, 66.

83. Escarce JJ, Jain AK, Rogowski J. Hospital competition, managed care, and mortality after hospitalization for medical conditions: evidence from three states. *Med Care Res Rev.* 2006;63(6 Suppl):112S–140S.

84. Rogowski J, Jain AK, Escarce JJ. Hospital competition, managed care, and mortality after hospitalization for medical conditions in California. *Health Serv Res.* 2007;42(2):682–705.

85. Bevan G, Skellern M. Does competition between hospitals improve clinical quality? A review of evidence from two eras of competition in the English NHS. *BMJ.* 2011;343:d6470.

86. Le Grand J. *The Other Invisible Hand: Delivering Public Services Through Choice and Competition.* Princeton, NJ: Princeton University Press; 2007.

87. Acute inpatient PPS. Centers for Medicare & Medicaid Services website. https://www.cms.gov/AcuteInpatientPPS/. Accessed November 20, 2011.

88. Shapiro MF, Park RE, Keesey J, Brook RH. The effect of alternative case-mix adjustments on mortality differences between municipal and voluntary hospitals in New York City. *Health Serv Res.* 1994;29(1):95–112.

89. Covinsky KE, Justice AC, Rosenthal GE, Palmer RM, Landefeld CS. Measuring prognosis and case mix in hospitalized elders: the importance of functional status. *J Gen Intern Med.* 1997;12(4):203–208.

90. Feigenbaum AV. Total quality control. *Harvard Business Review.* 1956;34(6):93–101.

91. Bingham RS, Juran JM. *Quality Control Handbook.* New York, NY: McGraw-Hill; 1962.

92. Juran J. *Juran's Quality Control Handbook.* New York, NY: McGraw-Hill; 1988.

93. Asubonteng P, McCleary KJ, Munchus G. The evolution of quality in the US health care industry: an old wine in a new bottle. *Int J Health Care Qual Assur.* 1996;9(3):11–19.

94. Harrington HJ. *Poor-Quality Cost.* New York, NY, and Milwaukee, WI: M. Dekker and ASQC Quality Press; 1987.

95. Deming WE. *On Probability as a Basis for Action.* Washington, DC: American Statistical Association; 1975.

96. Deming WE. *Out of the Crisis: Quality, Productivity and Competitive Position.* Cambridge, UK: Cambridge University Press; 1986.

97. NIST. Process or product monitoring and control. In: *NIST/SEMATECH e-Handbook of Statistical Methods.* Washington, DC: National Institute of Standards and Technology; 2006.

98. Neely YJA. Six Sigma—friend or foe? Cranfield University School of Management website. http://www.som.cranfield.ac.uk/som/dinamic-content/research/cbp/CBPupdate 1-SixSigmaFriendOrFoe.pdf. Accessed November 7, 2011.

99. Breen SL, Moseley DJ, Zhang B, Sharpe MB. Statistical process control for IMRT dosimetric verification. *Med Phys.* 2008;35(10):4417–4425.

100. Ettinger WH. Six Sigma: adapting GE's lessons to health care. *Trustee: The Journal For Hospital Governing Boards.* 2001;54(8):10.

101. Brigham EF, Daves PR. Capital budgeting: decision criteria. In: *Intermediate Financial Management.* 8th ed. 2004.

CHAPTER 8

Quantifying the Quality Performance Gaps

INTRODUCTION

The objective of this chapter is to lay out a strategic planning framework driven by organizational performance considerations. This framework is based on setting of performance targets and then identification of gaps between the current status and the performance targets. In contrast to the conventional finance-centered planning process, this framework will be driven not only by financial performance targets but also by quality performance targets. Thus, any strategy adopted will have to balance the financial and quality aspirations of the organization both in the short run and in the long run.

GOALS AND OBJECTIVES

After reading this chapter, the reader should be able to:

1. Define performance measurement.
2. Describe the process of performance measure selection.
3. Describe the relationship between financial performance and quality performance.
4. Describe the equilibrium between financial performance and quality performance.

5. Describe why and how organizations should assess their performance status.
6. Describe the role of an organization's values and mission in assessment of organizational performance.
7. Define the business case for quality.
8. Explain how performance targets could be set.

PERFORMANCE MEASUREMENT

As discussed previously in this text, it is helpful to have a good understanding of what is involved in the definition and achievement of organizational success. The next important step once success is envisioned is measurement; for without measurement, the organization will not know where it stands along the path to defined success. It may not even know how to communicate its vision of success to others. Therefore, this chapter will focus on measurement and quantification of performance expectations and performance gaps, which is necessary to communicate direction as well as distance to success.

The basic concepts of strategy and performance were previously introduced in this text, and the importance of finance and quality in organizational performance and success were reviewed. Performance measurement, not surprisingly, is often a poorly defined concept. Even if defined, the degree of variability involved in measurement of performance across a range of dimensions often makes organizational comparisons difficult. There exist models that have been used for measurement of performance in an organization with various dimensions of success, such as balanced scorecard,[1] performance prism,[2] and competing values framework.[3]

Lack of a clear definition of what constitutes a business performance measurement (BPM) system spans from features of such a system to its role and even its processes.[4] The roles of a BPM can be captured in one or more of the following[4]:

1. Performance measurement
2. Strategy management
3. Communication
4. Behavior modification
5. Learning and improvement

The process of creating a BPM is captured in the following categories[4]:

1. Selection/design of measures
2. Collection/manipulation of data
3. Information management
4. Performance evaluation
5. System review

It is important to reemphasize that *organizational performance* is not synonymous with *financial performance*. If there ever was a time that finance was the only focus for business executives, that era has long passed, and modern business executives need to (and often do) look beyond immediate financial goals.

There is no dispute that a *long-term* goal of businesses is financial viability, which in turn may have somewhat different meanings depending on the for-profit versus nonprofit nature of an organization. As the business environment has grown in its complexity and sophistication, the path to long-term success may go through long periods of shifting priorities for the organization. Such priorities all aim to secure the organization's future viability; these priorities may at times be at odds with financial objectives, but management recognizes that to win the war, it may have to lose a particular battle here and there.

By assuming such a position, management realizes that "enhanced competitiveness depends on starting from scratch and asking: 'Given our mission, what are the most important measures of performance?' 'How do these measures relate to one another?' 'What measures truly predict long-term financial success in our businesses?'"[5]

Decline in product quality while management had its eyes on the financial ball has been blamed for the eventual downturn in the financial performance of some businesses.[5] Today, the story of GM versus Toyota is common knowledge. Although this does not directly translate to medical care, local, regional, and national competition in health care is a fact of life today, and we are already seeing some international travel for medical care, the so-called medical tourism phenomenon.[6,7] For now, the main drivers are cost and value as defined earlier; in the future this may also include specific consideration of quality. As it is widely recognized that quality of health care is an important component of performance, two questions need to be answered:

1. How should quality be measured?
2. How can finance and quality be balanced?

Both of these questions can be answered by iterative processes similar to the eight-step process described for balanced scorecard[8] and are discussed further in the following paragraphs.

Measures, Indicators, and Metrics

As described previously in this text, a quality measure is defined as "a mechanism to assign a quantity to quality of care by comparison to a criterion."[9] This definition was expanded to define *measure* as a mechanism to assign a quantity to a variable of interest according to a criterion. This is to ensure consistency of definition across different aspects of organizational performance.

As described previously, an indicator is defined as a composite of measures grouped together according to a consensus. Subsequently, a quality metric was defined as a composite of quality indicators that represent a specific dimension of quality. In the context of this text, different aspects of healthcare quality are grouped under six main categories represented by the six aims (dimensions) introduced by the Institute of Medicine (IOM). Therefore, there will be six groups of quality indicators.

Finally, a performance metric is defined as a summary representation of a group of indicators that are closely related to a broad aspect of organizational performance, such as each of the six IOM aims for a group of operations (**Figure 8-1**).

The example of labeling medication bags with patient's name and medical record number was used to illustrate the grouping of measures into indicators and the use of indicators to create metrics. It must, however, be emphasized that the organization's management and board of directors will determine what indicators and metrics will best provide them with quality information they need.

Financial Performance Metrics

There exist multiple financial metrics for measurement of performance and to aid decision making during strategic planning. These metrics are strongly related to other financial indicators and to more subtle financial measures in a financial performance measurement system. As part of the discussion of interactions of finance and strategy, it is important to recognize the high-level financial metrics. Two of these, NPV and IRR methods, were discussed earlier in this text, and that discussion will not be repeated here. This context for organizational performance has evolved and has been refined over a long period of time. To a large extent, the treatment of quality performance has yet to go through a similar evolution and refinement.

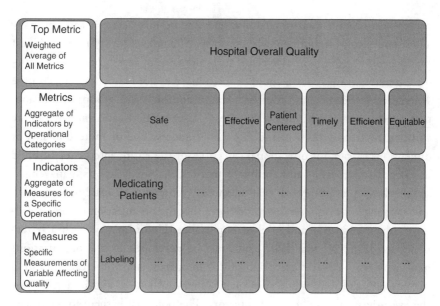

FIGURE 8-1. A hierarchical view of quality measures, indicators, and metrics. A metric corresponds to one or more of the IOM aims. An organization can create an aggregate value of the metrics as "top quality metric" and define it as appropriate to represent its quality performance level. Of course, boundaries have to be defined, and the metric must have true meaning. This will allow an organization to monitor periodically its performance with respect to quality.

Quality Performance Metrics

Like most other things in life, outcomes are the bottom line with respect to measurement of success along the path of quality improvement. However, without a careful analysis of the link between access, process, and structure of care, improvements in outcomes seem unattainable.

Fortunately, this important relationship has been recognized, and such relationships are being actively studied. Various government and nongovernment organizations are investigating a number of clinical (process) and organizational (structure) variables to determine their role in improvement of outcomes. The catch is that there are too many variables, and their weights in how they affect outcomes are different. Additionally, the ultimate net effect of modifying these variables is confounded by the prevalence, acuity, and natural course of different illnesses.

As a result, the organization that plans to include quality as a major performance metric must have a deep understanding of the related indicators and measures, its patient population, and its case-mix before it can optimally allocate its resources and deploy them to specific tasks. Quality measures must clearly be linked to modifiable elements in domains of access, process, or structure so that an intervention could be introduced as needed. As discussed in the "Measures, Indicators, and Metrics" section, indicators are groups of measures that are closely related under a domain or dimension of care, and metrics are constructed from groups of indicators that address one or more domains or dimensions of care for operational categories or the entire enterprise. To build the aggregate indicators and eventually metrics, the organization's management should develop a framework that adequately represents its patient population and the range of diagnoses and procedures that the organization covers according to their frequency and level of importance. Unfortunately, such a system is not available "off the shelf" and must be developed by the organization's management. Successful execution of this important step will create meaningful, reliable, and valid metrics for quality that can be used and understood by the executives and the board of directors. The potential is there for complexity and excessive detail in pursuit of this important aspect of organizational performance. Consequently, each organization will have to decide what areas within its clinical services will receive the highest priority and focus in building its quality performance system. To try to cover all areas with maximum detail will overwhelm the resources of the organization and therefore will defeat the overall purpose of introducing quality alongside finance as an important basis for organizational performance.

In addition to creation of aggregate metrics for the six IOM aims, a healthcare organization may create a top metric that is an aggregate of all quality metrics. To be meaningful, such a metric must represent the *weighted* sum of the IOM metrics and must be evaluated over time within the organization to ensure its reliability and validity in representing the aggregate level of quality within the organization. The weighting must also be determined according to the needs of the organization. For example, because safety has life and death consequences, it may carry more weight than efficiency. Organizations, depending on the population they serve and their for-profit, nonprofit, or government status, may have different priorities, which may be reflected in the weights they give to the six IOM aims.

An important caveat is that such a top metric will not be appropriate for comparison of one organization with another. Rather, it will be a measure of the internal state of quality and will serve to guide the organization's direction along its quality path. As such, it will be of use to board members and executives as part of the organization's navigation system. If properly linked to real-time data, this metric can be updated frequently and serve as one of the vital signs of the organization's own health. Should there be an unexpected change, management can trace back the source of the deviation and address it accordingly using drill down functions to get to lower level metrics, indicators, or even measures. The IOM metrics can also be treated the same way; however, at times a single metric may be more desirable than six.

Later in this text, organizational feedback and control will be discussed in more detail.

Determination of Measures of Performance

What to measure and how to measure are the key questions when it comes to measurement of performance. There exist multistep processes that add more detail on how this can be done, the most popular one being the balanced scorecard.[8,10]

Researchers suggest that the best approach would be to start with five generic measures: technical quality, customer satisfaction, speed, product cost reduction, and cash flow from operations, ensuring they are[11] (1) integrated, hierarchically and across business functions, and (2) based on a thorough understanding of the organization's cost drivers.

Upon closer examination of these five generic measures, one may conclude that these five actually belong to two broader categories of measures: financial measures (speed, product cost reduction, and cash flow from operations) and quality measures (technical quality, customer satisfaction). Of the two performance categories of finance and quality, the former has been the center of attention of executives and investors for a very long time. Therefore, the measures for financial performance have become well developed and accepted. In contrast, especially in health care, quality performance measures are still evolving. Fortunately, in recent years research in this area has picked up some momentum and has grown in sophistication.

From a practical point of view, quality measures must meet the general requirements of a business performance measure. Although this is a necessary condition, in the case of health care it is not sufficient; more is expected of a healthcare quality performance measure. To that end, the Agency for Healthcare Research and Quality has established a clearinghouse that evaluates proposed healthcare quality measures based on a set of requirements. This entity is called the National Quality Measure Clearinghouse, or NQMC.[9]

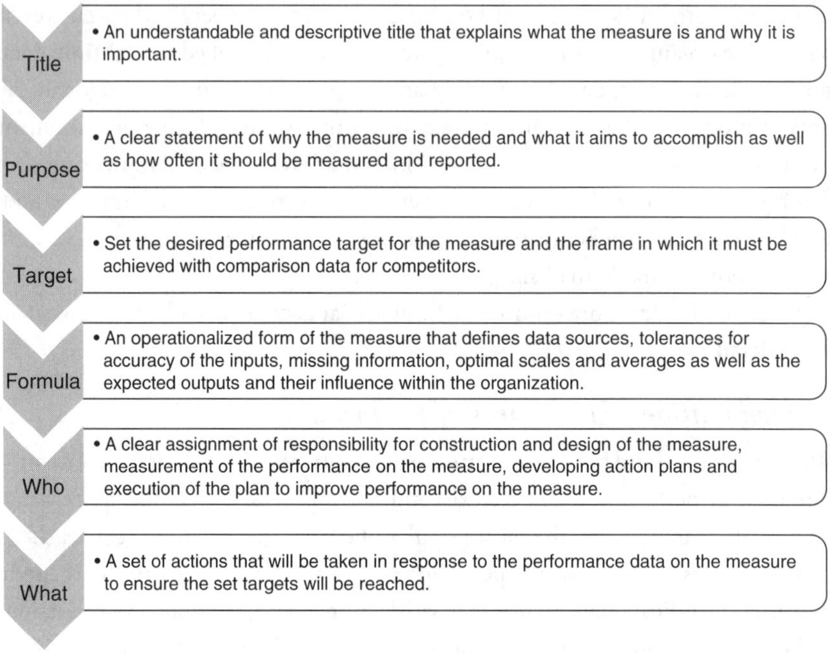

Title	• An understandable and descriptive title that explains what the measure is and why it is important.
Purpose	• A clear statement of why the measure is needed and what it aims to accomplish as well as how often it should be measured and reported.
Target	• Set the desired performance target for the measure and the frame in which it must be achieved with comparison data for competitors.
Formula	• An operationalized form of the measure that defines data sources, tolerances for accuracy of the inputs, missing information, optimal scales and averages as well as the expected outputs and their influence within the organization.
Who	• A clear assignment of responsibility for construction and design of the measure, measurement of the performance on the measure, developing action plans and execution of the plan to improve performance on the measure.
What	• A set of actions that will be taken in response to the performance data on the measure to ensure the set targets will be reached.

FIGURE 8-2. Measure design process.
Source: Adapted from Neely et al.[12]

To develop a properly and fully operationalized performance measure, a process must be in place. There are many such processes described in the literature, and one that has the most relevant features is presented here[12] (**Figure 8-2**).

Selected measures must be clearly defined and owned. The link between the measure, related outcomes, and consequences of success and failure with respect to the measure must be firmly understood. Finally, intervention with respect to the measure must be possible.[12]

Linking Financial and Quality Performances

When quality measures are selected and incorporated into the performance model for an organization's quality, an estimate of the impact of the measures on other performance indicators for the organization is useful in the evaluation of the remedial actions necessary for overall performance. Although this will establish a link between quality and finance, it does not necessarily mean that the financial bottom line will dictate the course of action. Rather, it means that management will be able to foresee the consequences of the alternative actions and determine the most cost-effective alternative given the conditions in the business environment. In other words, a value can be quantified for quality that can help with decision making; there is supporting evidence in the literature for the usefulness of such efforts.[13]

This is not dissimilar to the conflicts between marketing and finance[14] and should be resolved in a similar fashion.

Equilibrium of Finance and Quality in the Strategic Plan

With the recognition of the bidirectional link between quality and finance in a healthcare organization, it follows that any changes to one can have an echo in the other. To determine the net result of a change in overall performance status of the organization, one must determine the point where the results of echoes will reach equilibrium. This state of equilibrium will give a much more accurate picture of the organization's performance status as a result of a strategy, and alternatives could be evaluated more rigorously.

To implement such a model, the consequences of strategic adjustments to affect quality performance on the organization's financial performance must be determined along with any potential feedback that might affect quality performance. The opposite is also true in the case of changes made that affect financial performance that in turn may have consequences on quality and subsequent feedback to financial performance.

The following example will illustrate this effect. Suppose that due to a difficult economic environment, an organization decides to reduce its nursing staff to save cost and improve the bottom line. If such an action results in deterioration of quality (increased medication errors or increased rate of preventable mishaps), quality may decline, and the organization will likely lose more in nonpayment from the payers than it will save. This in turn will further jeopardize the financial bottom line resulting in further decline in quality. Overall, this will have been a bad decision. However, if a decrease in nursing staff is judicious or is coupled with other measures that ensure maintenance of the quality level (through technology or other less expensive alternatives), the effect on quality may be negligible, making the move strategically sound.

Although the implications of this example may appear obvious, similar dynamics in more complex situations may well be overlooked during the planning process. Hence, the point of this text is that in very much the same way that the financial impact of any strategic decision is measured, the quality impact of any such decision must also be considered.

ASSESSMENT OF CURRENT QUALITY PERFORMANCE STATUS

Assessment of quality involves assessment of access, process, structure, outcomes, and patient experience.[15,16] For practical purposes, the IOM's definition of quality and the six related aims are appropriate areas that deserve primary focus.[17] It is incumbent upon management to systematically examine the quality of care delivered within the organization with respect to those six dimensions using instruments that are valid and reliable. Other characteristics of such an instrument are listed in Figure 8-2.

Other elements in quality will come to light when one looks at the processes in terms of overuse, underuse, and misuse.[18] Evaluation of error and defect rates in the organization by auditing processes will also reveal valuable information about quality of care delivered. These are different vantage points that provide invaluable information that could be used to address the underlying causes of the observed effects.

Useful indicators that reflect performance in each of those areas must be identified and validated by the management and then processed into relevant and clear quality indicators on the dashboard or quality report card. This is an incremental process and should always be considered as a work in progress given that the flow of new discoveries and treatments is a fact of life in health care. A measurement framework that consists of measures, indicators, and metrics with respect to organizations operations, as well as domains and dimensions of quality, was discussed elsewhere in the text. This framework must be implemented in conjunction with a performance presentation and reporting framework to enable the organization access to performance data as shown in **Figure 8-3**.

Insight into an Organization's Standing on the Quality Scale

A well-designed quality performance measurement system is not only able to identify and report variances but also is useful in identifying contributing causes. Management must prioritize the variances and problems in terms of their impact on mortality, morbidity, financial bottom line, and other factors that affect the overall effectiveness of the organization in provision of quality care and then initiate corrective action to address the problems.

Focusing of efforts on quality and quality improvement in a healthcare organization requires the broad participation of the rank and file of the organization. The only way to ensure that the organization as a whole is appreciative of and sensitive to the quality of care it provides would be to engage all parties involved.

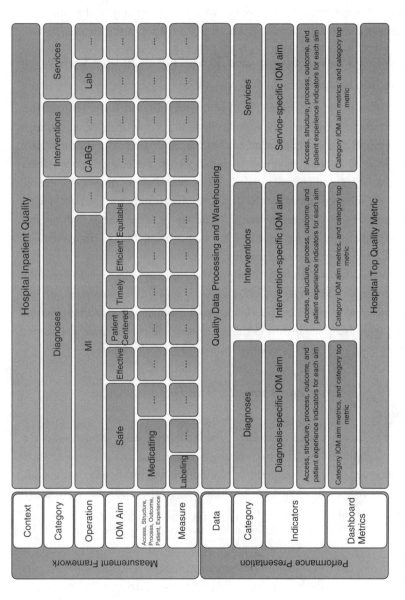

FIGURE 8-3. The quality measurement framework must have a matching framework for presentation and reporting of the performance data. Only then can the collected data be used to calculate composite metrics for each of the six IOM aims and even a single metric of quality if the organization so chooses.

There is evidence in the literature that active participation of nurses may play a significant role in improvement of outcome, potentially at no additional cost.[19]

Lower levels will be concerned with what happens in their own domains, but executives and boards must be involved in *all* aspects of quality in the same way they are concerned with the overall financial performance of the organization.

Reconciling Values, Mission, and Vision with Quality Status of the Organization

Values and mission are the foundation of an organization's identity. They are the fundamental motivation and clarity of purpose that constantly guide all employees and members of the organization toward the same goals. The organization's vision, which management wants all to participate in achieving, is constructed on a foundation of values and mission. These foundational principles should provide a clear message as to what the organization's attitude and purpose is with respect to the quality of care it delivers. It would not be surprising to find that the employees of many healthcare organizations are not aware of the values, mission, or vision of their respective organizations.[20]

For an organization effectively to improve the quality of care it delivers, not only is it necessary to reconcile the values, mission, and vision statements with the organization's quality status and goals, but also it is imperative that all employees be familiar with these statements, as the statements will provide a valuable sense of direction to employees in the daily performance of their duties.

Beyond Regulatory Requirements: The Business Case for Quality

It is possible that an organization may satisfy the regulatory requirements for quality. It may even be possible that the organization may not perceive any real quality threats vis-à-vis its competitors. Should the organization continue with its quality improvement initiatives? Should it set goals beyond what is *required*? How can the investment be justified?

If a healthcare organization seeks to improve its quality of care beyond the minimum requirements, both regulatory and competitive, then expecting a return on the investment in that improvement would seem logical. This expectation and associated results have been studied, and consequently, a "business case" for quality has emerged.

A business case for a healthcare quality improvement intervention exists if the organization realizes a financial return on the investment required for the intervention in a reasonable time frame using a reasonable rate of discounting. This return may be in the form of profits, reduction in losses, or avoided costs. A business case may also exist if the organization believes that a positive indirect effect on its function and sustainability will accrue within a reasonable time frame.[21]

One of the most influential forces in the healthcare quality movement is, no doubt, the payment system. In order for healthcare organizations to provide higher-quality care, they must make specified investments and commitments. Where chronic diseases and third-party payers are involved, the benefits of these investments might not accrue directly to the healthcare organization making those commitments. A deliberate study of the current environment and the mechanisms by which quality improvement efforts can potentially be rewarded or punished is a topic that involves all parties in the U.S. healthcare system, but more importantly, it involves the payers and policy makers.

Pay-for-performance is an attempt at aligning the incentives between payers and providers, including healthcare organizations, to adopt quality-enhancing interventions. This applies especially where there may exist a negative business case for quality from the perspective of the provider; however, the payer may benefit from the intervention. In these circumstances, a business case can be made if the sum of these two effects is positive. Consequently, a pay-for-performance agreement can be made between the payer and the provider, and therefore the intervention can be adopted.[22] It is imperative to understand that for such arguments to be made, the costs of quality-enhancing interventions, including investment and operating costs of implementation as well as the changes in revenue and costs that result from the interventions, must be carefully tracked and projected.[23,24]

ESTABLISHING QUALITY PERFORMANCE TARGETS

The first priority after identifying the measures and developing the indicators and performance metrics that will be used to declare success or failure is to review the organization's standing for each and every one of the quality indicators selected. This will establish the point of origin from which the organization hopes to advance.

The next step is to establish targets. The usual exercises of selection of targets as part of any strategic planning process apply here as well. Targets must be derived from an organization's mission and be relevant to its vision. The targets must take into account a realistic application of an organization's capabilities and must also recognize (and exploit) the opportunities that the organization faces. Finally, they must also realistically acknowledge the internal weaknesses and external threats facing the organization.

Overreaching targets that are incompatible with an organization's capabilities will only serve to disappoint or frustrate, and setting of too modest a target will result in an organization falling far short of its potential. Therefore, a thorough exercise in analysis of strengths, weaknesses, opportunities, and threats (SWOT analysis) is essential. In addition, the quality targets must be reviewed in light of their impact on overall outcomes indicators such as mortality. This is one way that management can prioritize where it wants to allocate resources. Synergistic interactions among targets must also be examined.

The organization will have to be cognizant of at least three distinct levels for quality performance, or any other performance metric for that matter. The first level (A) is the minimum requirement as set by regulations or otherwise below which there is no point in remaining in the business. The second important level (B) is where an organization's competitors in that market stand and their relative distance to where the organization is. The third level (C) is where the organization's ideals picture it to be. Thinking in these terms will allow the organization's board and management to find a sense of direction by surpassing the minimum requirements, setting their posture relative to competition, and moving toward the ideal. This process, often referred to as *positioning,* is central to the long-term viability of the organization.

When the current state is determined and targets are set, the gaps will determine the time frame and resources needed to undertake the tasks that will result in achieving the targets. Once the organization has identified its current position and determines its existing (and desired) relative position to the competition, it can position itself in the community or marketplace. In many industries, quality (a subtype of differentiation) is one of the three generic recipes for success, the other two being cost leadership and focus.[25] This may be different in health care, as it is not clear whether the informed consumer will choose lower quality over cost. A safer strategy would be to match or surpass the competition while containing cost by way of improved productivity. At times, circumstances may necessitate matching or surpassing the competition even at greater cost in the short term, although unless this is coupled with increased productivity or other cost recovery measures over the long term, this strategy will not be sustainable. **Figure 8-4** depicts these dynamics.

In looking at Figure 8-4, the reader is cautioned against simply considering productivity as a function of outputs given the inputs of the organization. An instance of this definition that is most widely used by healthcare organizations

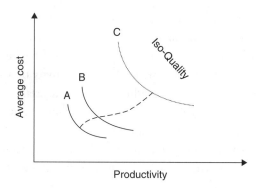

FIGURE 8-4. Relationship between quality, cost, and productivity. A, B, and C are iso-quality curves plotting organizations that deliver the same quality of care at different average costs. The higher the cost, the lower the productivity. The dashed line denotes a path to improvement of quality that is coupled with an increase in productivity.

uses the number of encounters, discharges, or patients served as the output. This interpretation of output in this definition is a narrow one at best and can be misleading. To measure productivity properly, quality must be factored in when output is measured.

To demonstrate the flaw in the above definition, consider a hospital that serves n patients per year, with a cumulative mortality and morbidity rate of m. This hospital finds out that by cutting certain costs, it can serve the same n patients per year at a 5% reduction in its use of resources (i.e., at 95% input). The drawback is an increase in cumulative mortality and morbidity rate. Using the common instance of the definition (i.e., number of patients n served per year over input), one can show an increase in productivity (**Equation 8-1**).

$$P_0 = \frac{n}{\text{input}} \Rightarrow P_1 \frac{n}{0.95 \times \text{input}}$$

Equation 8-1. Increased productivity P as a result of a reduction in input.

However, this comes at a cost: decreased quality. It must be emphasized that oftentimes, such changes are not linked to changes in quality. It is, therefore, appropriate and even necessary to consider the role of quality in measurement of productivity.

By looking at Figure 8-4, one can see that different organizations that share a similar quality performance level will fall on a curve plotted against average cost and productivity. Achieving a higher level of quality for one organization would mean moving from one curve to the next one. Depending on an organization's strategy, this could result in increased average cost (the y axis will represent incremental average cost) at the same level of productivity or a smaller increase in cost if combined with increased productivity. In rare instances, it may even be possible to have no increase in cost by simply improving productivity and at the same time achieving a higher level of quality.

Other factors that influence these curves and movement from one to another include cost recovery strategies, competition, and time frame envisioned for the change.

REFERENCES

1. Kaplan RS, Norton DP. The balanced scorecard—measures that drive performance. *Harvard Business Review.* 1992;70(1):71–79.
2. Neely A, Adams C. The performance prism perspective. *Journal of Cost Management.* 2001;15(1):7.
3. Wicks AM, St. Clair L. Competing values in healthcare: balancing the (un)balanced scorecard. *J Healthc Manag.* 2007;52(5):309–324.
4. Franco-Santos M, Kennerley M, Micheli P, et al. Towards a definition of a business performance measurement system. *International Journal of Operations and Production Management.* 2007;27(8):784–801.
5. Eccles RG. The performance measurement manifesto. *Harvard Business Review.* 1991;69(1):131–137.
6. Brown SB. Datapage. Medical tourism: nations vie for health dollars. *Hosp Health Netw.* 2008;82(12):49.
7. Horowitz MD, Rosensweig JA, Jones CA. Medical tourism: globalization of the healthcare marketplace. *MedGenMed.* 2007;9(4):33.
8. Kaplan RS, Norton DP. Putting the balanced scorecard to work. *Harvard Business Review.* 1993;71(5):134–147.
9. Child health care quality toolbox: understanding quality measurement. Agency for Healthcare Research and Quality website. http://www.ahrq.gov/chtoolbx/understn .htm#whata. Published 2004. Accessed November 4, 2011.
10. Wisner JD, Fawcett SE. Linking firm strategy to operating decisions through performance measurement. *Production & Inventory Management Journal.* 1991;32(3):5–11.
11. Keegan DP, Eiler RG, Jones CR. Are your performance measures obsolete? *Management Accounting.* 1989;70(12 June):45–50.
12. Adapted from Neely A, Bourne M, Kennerley M. Dysfunctional performance through dysfunctional measures. *Journal of Cost Management.* 2003;17(5):41–45.
13. Taylor R, Manzo J, Sinnett M. Quantifying value for physician order-entry systems: a balance of cost and quality. *Healthcare Financial Management.* 2002;56(7):44.
14. Barwise P, Marsh PR, Wensley R. Must finance and strategy clash? *Harvard Business Review.* 1989;67(5):85–90.
15. Donabedian A. Evaluating the quality of medical care. *Milbank Mem Fund Q.* 1966; 44(3, Suppl):166–206.

16. Domain framework and inclusion criteria. Agency for Healthcare Research and Quality website http://www.qualitymeasures.ahrq.gov/about/domain-definitions.aspx. Accessed November 5, 2011.

17. Committee on Quality of Health Care in America. *Crossing the Quality Chasm: A New Health System for the 21st Century.* Washington, DC: Institute of Medicine; 2001.

18. Chassin MR. Is health care ready for Six Sigma quality? *Milbank Q.* 1998;76(4): 565–591, 510.

19. Khatri N, Baveja A, Boren SA, Mammo A. Medical errors and quality of care: from control to commitment. *California Management Review.* 2006;48(3):115–141.

20. Desmidt S, Heene A. Mission statement perception: are we all on the same wavelength? A case study in a Flemish hospital. *Health Care Manag Rev.* 2007;32(1): 77–87.

21. Leatherman S, Berwick D, Iles D, et al. The business case for quality: case studies and an analysis. *Health Aff (Millwood).* 2003;22(2):17–30.

22. Wheeler JRC, White B, Rauscher S, et al. Pay-for-performance as a method to establish the business case for quality. *Journal of Health Care Finance.* 2007;33(4):17–30.

23. Kilpatrick KE, Lohr KN, Leatherman S, et al. The insufficiency of evidence to establish the business case for quality. *Int J Qual Health Care.* 2005;17(4):347–355.

24. Fetterolf D, West R. The business case for quality: combining medical literature research with health plan data to establish value for nonclinical managers. *Am J Med Qual.* 2004;19(2):48–55.

25. Porter ME. Generic competitive strategies. In: *Competitive Strategy: Techniques for Analyzing Industries and Competitors.* New York, NY: The Free Press; 1980:34–46.

Closing the Gaps

INTRODUCTION

Earlier chapters developed a path to guide a healthcare organization toward understanding and envisioning its definition of success while also communicating this perspective to all stakeholders. Once an organization has successfully measured its current performance and has decided where it wants to be with respect to those performance measures, it should begin a planning process to develop a strategy to achieve its goals. This chapter will address the process for strategy development as well as strategy monitoring to ensure that during its journey, the organization will be in a position to make course corrections as necessary.

GOALS AND OBJECTIVES

After reading this chapter, the reader should be able to:

1. Define *performance-driven planning*.
2. Apply a strengths, weaknesses, opportunities, and threats (SWOT) analysis to determine performance gaps.
3. Identify solutions to close performance gaps based on SWOT analysis.
4. Discuss the concept of aligning the incentives with quality.
5. Describe the different categories of strategies with respect to quality of care.
6. Describe the role of economics in healthcare quality and strategy development.

7. Describe the concepts of cost-effectiveness analysis and comparative effectiveness research and their application as important tools for strategy development.
8. Define the feedback control of the quality improvement strategy performance.
9. Describe a high-level organizational performance dashboard and the appropriate information it should display.

PERFORMANCE-DRIVEN PLANNING

Although there may be many past writings that provide a rationale and underlying basis for the concept of "performance-driven planning," perhaps the two most notable from a historical perspective are Avedis Donabedian's 1966 seminal article on medical care quality[1] and "Habit 2: Begin with the End in Mind," a chapter in Stephen Covey's influential 1989 book.[2]

Avedis Donabedian, whom many regard as the father of the modern understanding of quality in medical care, presented a paradigm for conceptualizing quality in medical care. His three-domain paradigm of structure, process, and outcome,[1] now expanded to include access and patient experience,[3] provides a framework for the description of healthcare quality at any level, whether for a small office or a national healthcare system.

At the level of a healthcare system, *access* refers to the availability of a service (in this case health care) to a patient or a group of patients. *Structure* refers to the characteristics and attributes of the settings and of the personnel delivering the care (capacity, technology, licensing, credentialing, etc.). *Process* refers to the practices that are followed in the provision of care (standards, protocols, pathways, etc.). *Outcome* refers to the results achieved from the delivery of care (patient health and functional status). *Patient experience* refers to the patient's assessment of the quality of care he or she has received. Clearly, these five domains are related and connected (**Figure 9-1**). Moreover, the first three (access, structure, and process) can be directly modified, whereas the outcome cannot. Patient experience although modifiable is subjective and may be influenced by factors that do not affect the outcome.

It is a relatively small leap to take the domains of this paradigm and apply them to organizational characteristics. In fact, it seems particularly appropriate to apply this framework to healthcare organizations. *Access* is whether patients

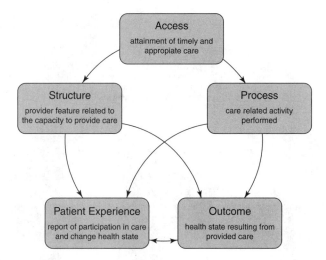

FIGURE 9-1. The relationship between the modified Donabedian domains of quality. Measures in any of these domains could relate to one or more IOM aims, or dimensions of quality. Arrows depict how measures in each domain may influence other domains.

who meet the indication for a medical intervention can receive it and is related to availability of the intervention at the appropriate time or location and the patient's ability to pay through a variety of sources. In the absence of universal coverage, access is an important issue. However, even with universal coverage, access remains an issue; for example, living in a remote area would still be a barrier to ensuring access. *Structure* refers to the organizational design, or the organizational "chart," of functions, reporting relationships, responsibilities, authority, and so forth. *Process* refers to the organizational activities, initiatives under way, programs, and actions being taken. *Outcome* refers to the results and performance achieved by the organization. Finally, *patient experience* reflects the patient's satisfaction with the care he or she has received. Describing the organization in terms of these five domains at some future point in time can also serve as one approach to characterizing the organization's "vision" at that future point in time.

Given the Donabedian paradigm as applied to organizations and bringing in Covey's notion of "begin with the end in mind," the rationale for performance-driven planning becomes self-evident. This seemingly backward approach simply calls for setting outcome and performance targets (goals and expectations) beginning with the end in mind, and then formulating initiatives and actions

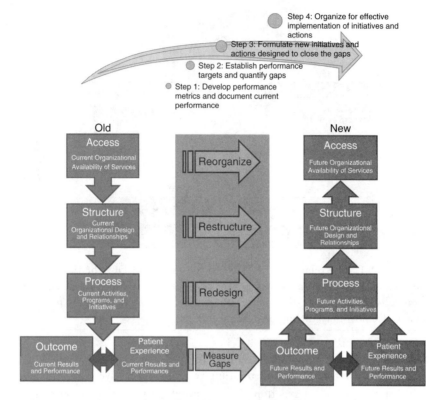

FIGURE 9-2. Moving from the old access–structure–process–outcome–patient experience model to the new outcome (and patient experience)–process (and access)–structure (and access) model through performance-driven planning.

(processes) that can serve as a bridge to take the organization from its current performance to its desired performance; that is, the end in mind (**Figure 9-2**).

The organization is designed (structured) to best enable implementation of the formulated initiatives to achieve the targeted or desired outcomes (performance). As the organization engages in this approach to the planning process, the first stage in which the measures, indicators, and metrics of performance are defined must be viewed as the construction of the "navigational system." These metrics will form the basis for judging the acceptability and contribution of any proposed initiative; that is, what that proposed initiative will contribute toward the achievement of the targeted performance and, hence, the gap closure. In this respect, each performance gap should be evaluated in terms of the strengths, weaknesses, opportunities, and threats (SWOT) analysis directly related to that gap. Without these "gap-defining" indicators and metrics clearly established as the basis for selection of strategic initiatives, charting of the organizational path will be very much like flying without a navigational system and a destination in mind. It is critical to ensure that the selected performance metrics are not arbitrarily chosen; rather, they are derived from mission and based on the notion of mission accountability (i.e., how will the organization's performance with respect to mission be judged).

Identifying Gap-Related Issues: SWOT Analysis

Once goals (targets) have been set and the differences between current performance and those goals (targets) are identified, the next step is development of a plan to close the gaps. The SWOT analysis (specific to each gap) referred to earlier is helpful in capitalizing on the organization's strengths and exploiting the potential opportunities while at the same time taking into account the organization's internal weaknesses and external threats.

It is also important to recognize that instances of the four elements of a SWOT analysis can vary significantly depending on an organization's orientation, size, and geography.[4] From the perspective of a health care organization, depending on where they stand on the quality of care they provide, quality considerations and implications may be present in any of the four SWOT groups. For instance, a competitor with a higher quality of care may pose a threat not only because it is a competitor in general but also because it specifically provides higher quality care.

Each healthcare organization should analyze its internal and external environment in terms of the framework of a SWOT analysis to be able to assess its relative competitive status and put forward strategies to survive and to compete.

Developing Initiatives and Interventions to Close the Gaps

After a SWOT analysis specific to the gaps identified earlier is performed, strategies could be devised and initiatives proposed to close the gaps by addressing the findings of the analysis. These strategies must be compatible with an organization's values and are guided by its mission. After ensuring consistency with the organization's values and mission, the strategic feasibility of the initiatives is evaluated.

In general (as described earlier), this will be followed by determination of operational feasibility and, finally, financial feasibility. As a result, unless the initiative is specifically aimed at dealing with some aspect of healthcare quality, its impact on the quality of care delivered by the organization will not come to light until much later, if ever. Considering quality as an integral part of any strategy (similar to finance), any negative or positive effect of the initiative on the quality of care delivered must be considered during the SWOT analysis and during the early development phase. After all, quality is a strategic weapon[5] and can be an internal strength or weakness, a competitive threat posed to the organization by its competitors, or an opportunity for the organization relative to its competitors.

Operational and financial feasibility studies complete the evaluation process, and management can then decide which strategy or initiative to adopt. Inclusion of considerations of the impact of the proposed strategy or initiative on the quality of care would enhance the evaluation process. Indeed, with appropriate analysis, quality of care improvement could be used to make projections about its impact on financial measures thus enhancing the ability of management to have a more comprehensive view of the potential end results.

INTEGRATION OF FINANCE AND QUALITY

Whether it is because quality of care is demanded by the consumer, required by the payer, mandated by the regulatory bodies, or deficient with respect to quality performance in other industries, it has become a focus of attention in health care. The pressure is mounting to the point where quality can no longer be a secondary concern and simply treated with occasional quality-enhancing initiatives and ad hoc tactical moves. Quality of care should be treated as a pervasive measure of performance throughout the organization. In addition to its financial impact, every initiative and proposal should be evaluated in terms of its impact on improving the quality standing and health of the organization. For this to happen, carefully designed quality performance measures must also be studied with respect to their potential financial footprint—positive, neutral, or negative. Management teams should pursue and build business cases for initiatives that will improve quality significantly and seek partnerships with payers in this pursuit. From a broader perspective, policy makers should allow and encourage such efforts that would contribute to enhanced financial viability of healthcare organizations.

The financial impact of poor quality on healthcare organizations and the healthcare industry is substantial. The potential savings resulting from a reduction in the number of preventable injuries or deaths (medical errors) is a staggering figure. Discovery of strategies that allow this cost to be spent on the delivery of health care rather than on dealing with the consequences of poor-quality health care will certainly prove to be cost-effective in the long run. To accomplish this, access and structures need to be modified, processes changed, and policies updated.

Although this may sound idealistic, it remains true that quality should be as pervasive an organizational performance metric as is finance. The priority of every strategy adopted by any healthcare organization has been to contribute to the competitiveness and financial viability (short term or long term) of the organization. If the organization is not financially viable, its very survival, and therefore its mission, is at risk. Quality of care delivered in the healthcare industry has reached an equal level of importance.

Aligning Incentives for Quality: Opportunities and Threats

As discussed earlier, the payer–provider relationship historically has not been supportive of costly quality improvement efforts. Pay-for-performance (P4P), or value-based purchasing (VBP), has emerged as a way of incentivizing providers by splitting the financial gains that payers may enjoy if the providers have better outcomes or meet certain quality standards.[6] This is a new effort, and there are no long-term data showing how successful it has been. In a review of the literature on the P4P effect on quality of health care, researchers found evidence for positive effects on quality measures.[7] This, however, is not supported by a more recent study looking into the effects of P4P on outcomes of acute myocardial infarction. In this study, the authors were not able to detect positive or negative effects of P4P on the outcomes.[8] Other studies into core measures and P4P have also found no link between outcomes and P4P.[9,10]

In order for P4P to have a positive and lasting effect on quality of care, it should be aimed at the proper quality measures and indicators, and it should allow for a business case to be made for the providers, in particular, healthcare organizations. Healthcare organizations must also be diligent in identifying their quality challenges and make a business case for quality improvement based on monetary and nonmonetary effects of such improvements. Healthcare organizations should also consider negotiating P4P arrangements with payers. They must realize that although P4P functions as a threat, in it one might also find opportunities.

It is not clear how long the incentives must remain in place and what will happen when the differentiation based on performance linked to incentives is lost.[11] Equally unclear are the unintended side effects of such incentives; for instance, providers that exclude sicker patients who may adversely affect their outcomes.[12] It is also not clear whether P4P can ultimately bring down the rising cost of health care.[13] Others have argued that in the end, higher quality of care would result in lower costs by eliminating excesses and waste in the healthcare system.[11]

Two major driving forces behind an organization's strategic agenda for quality improvement are the regulatory environment and competition. Considering these two forces, one can classify various strategies that improve the quality

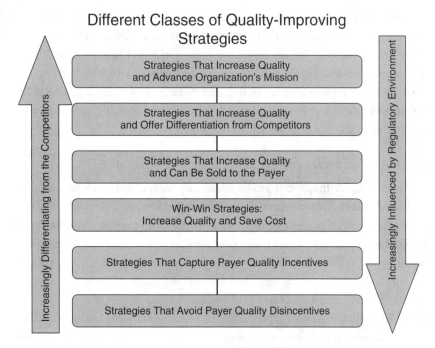

FIGURE 9-3. A hierarchical view of different types or classes of strategies that can result in improvements in the quality of care that is delivered in a healthcare organization.

of care delivered in an organization into six distinct classes (**Figure 9-3**). A brief description of this classification is presented in the following paragraphs.

Avoid Payer Disincentives

The most reactive strategy would be simply to avoid the losses incurred as a result of payer disincentives. For example, Medicare will not reimburse hospitals for preventable complications of inpatient care such as decubitus ulcers and catheter-related infections. By preventing these complications, the organization will avoid financial losses as a result of disincentives and at the same time improve quality.

Capture Payer Incentives

Next in the hierarchy is the somewhat less reactive strategy of capturing payer incentives. As discussed previously, the VBP program by CMS will reduce DRG payments by 1% in 2013 and 2% by 2017. These savings will be used to fund incentive payments to hospitals that meet a set of designated standards.[14]

Capturing these incentives while improving quality of care is a sound strategy for a health care organization.

Save Cost and Increase Quality

This is the first stage in the development of proactive strategies. There are scenarios where an increase in quality will benefit both the payer and the organization. For example, avoiding preventable complications from medication errors may result in cost savings for the hospital, increase quality of care delivered, and also save money for payers as they no longer have to cover the costs of dealing with those complications. Venous thromboembolism (VTE) prophylaxis is another example. Ensuring that every patient admitted to the hospital is assessed for his or her risk of development of VTE and taking proper prophylactic action is an important step in avoiding costs associated with a hospital-acquired condition.[15]

Strategies That Can Be Sold to the Payer

This is a somewhat more proactive strategy. The organization may identify quality improvement measures that will reduce a payer's cost but will not improve the organization's financial bottom line and in fact may negatively affect it. If the payer's savings are more than the organization's losses, a business case can be made to the payer to split the savings. Such an arrangement will create a win–win situation where (1) quality of care is improved, (2) the payer reduces its costs (but not quite as much), and (3) the organization may improve its financial bottom line.

Differentiation from Competition

Although also proactive, this is a risky (returns not guaranteed) proposition requiring creativity and a lot of thought. This may be costly in the short run, but, assuming that appropriate and valid public reporting mechanisms for quality performance are in place, the organization will (1) be more appealing to the consumer, (2) be able to bargain with the payers, and (3) force the competition also to improve its quality. The end result will certainly favor higher-quality organizations. However, organizations that take the initiative in differentiating themselves from competitors in quality must not lose sight of the continuing need for efficiency and long-term financial viability.

Adherence to Mission

The last of the six classes describes the most altruistic of the strategies: remaining true to the organization's mission at all cost, assuming the organization's mission includes high-quality care. This strategy, although principled and noble, can only be viable if innovative measures to increase efficiency and quality are combined to ensure the long-term financial viability of the organization. If successful, this strategy has the added benefit of differentiating the organization from its competition.

Economics of Quality

Two of the six Institute of Medicine (IOM) aims, effectiveness and efficiency, directly affect financial performance and the economics of care. There are important points to be made about efficacy—a prerequisite to determination of effectiveness of care in an evidenced-based healthcare environment—effectiveness, and efficiency.

Efficacy in health care most commonly refers to the ability of a treatment (medication or intervention) to do more good than harm.[16] Efficacy has to do with meeting of the targets and therefore is used mostly in clinical trials. The question about a treatment most commonly asked with respect to efficacy is "Can it work?"[16]

Effectiveness, in contrast, has to do with the question "Does it work?"[16] This is a reflection of the fact that if a treatment works under the restrictive (ideal) conditions of a clinical trial, it may not actually have the same success in actual clinical use. As expected for an intervention to be part of the standard of care, it must be effective. Subsequent to this determination is the question of cost of the intervention. It is certainly desirable to opt for a less costly and equally effective intervention should more than one option be available. This is the subject matter of cost-effectiveness analysis.

Efficiency is a term used in different ways across the various branches of science. When used in a healthcare context, the term most commonly refers to productive or technical efficiency. Productive efficiency requires expending only the minimum required resources to produce a given level of product[17] or, in this context, outcome.

The three most widely used methods of economic evaluation are cost-effectiveness analysis (CEA), cost utility analysis (CUA), and cost benefit analysis (CBA).

CEA compares a single, common effect in terms of cost among two or more alternatives. This effect, life years gained, units of weight lost, and so forth, may be achieved to different degrees by different alternatives.[16]

CUA compares single or multiple effects that are not necessarily common among two or more alternatives. These effects are typically measured in quality adjusted life years (QALYs). In one single measure, QALYs capture the gains from reduced morbidity (quality) and the gains from reduced mortality (quantity).[16] This makes them very useful in comparing two or more interventions that address the same illness; for example, kidney transplant versus lifelong hemodialysis. CUA and CEA are synonymous in the U.S. literature.

CBA compares single or multiple effects that are not necessarily common among two or more alternatives. Benefits are measured in monetary units, and as expected, it may be difficult to measure all benefits of alternative programs in monetary units. In contrast, if most benefits are measured in monetary units, a CBA can determine if a program is worthwhile.[16] CBA is not very relevant to evaluation of treatment options or clinical trials. Rather, it is an important assessment tool in public health and policy decisions.

As mentioned earlier, in health care, treatments (medications or interventions) are evaluated through clinical trials to determine their efficacy. After passage of the Kefauver–Harris Amendments in 1962, this became a legal requirement for U.S. Food and Drug Administration (FDA) approval. Almost 47 years later in 2009, the shortcomings of efficacy in evaluation of treatment options in clinical trials has been recognized. Comparative effectiveness research is hoped to look into the effectiveness and efficiency of interventions.

Competition and demand, two other important economic concepts that affect quality, were discussed previously in this text and will not be repeated here. To close the discussion of economics of quality, two important tools of economic evaluation of available alternatives, CEA and comparative effectiveness research, both of which have direct implications in planning, will be briefly reviewed here.

Cost Effectiveness and Efficiency in Quality Improvement Planning

In general terms, for a CEA to be relevant, alternatives must exist that may potentially have different costs or outcomes. Then, healthcare organizations can determine how best to achieve the desired outcome at a lower cost. In the simplest form, a CEA works as follows: (1) interventions must be able to achieve the desired effect, and (2) interventions with the lowest incremental cost per unit of effect will be the most cost-effective solution.

To apply CEA to quality improvement planning will imply that the organization knows how to achieve that level of quality and that it has more than one way to get there. CEA is an important tool in resource allocation and would allow management to prioritize its action plans and be more efficient. The Centers for Medicare & Medicaid Services (CMS) also advocates such analyses in dealing with quality improvement initiatives.[18]

Comparative Effectiveness Research

The American Recovery and Reinvestment Act of 2009 has provisioned $1.1 billion for comparative effectiveness research (CER).[19] Pursuant to this legislation, on March 19, 2009, the U.S. Department of Health and Human Services (HHS) announced the creation of a Federal Council for Comparative Effectiveness Research.[20,21] According to HHS:

> Comparative effectiveness research provides information on the relative strengths and weakness of various medical interventions. Such research will give clinicians and patients valid information to make decisions that will improve the performance of the U.S. health care system.[20]

The main idea behind this effort is to improve outcomes and curtail wasteful spending on healthcare interventions that fail to show comparative advantage over alternative interventions.[22–24] The true impact and success or failure of this effort will probably not be revealed for years. However, it will be worthwhile to promote a culture of efficiency in a healthcare organization by promoting consideration of available alternatives in diagnostic workups and treatment plans. This is an area that has been lacking and may soon be under scrutiny.[23,24]

Comparative effectiveness aims at providing more and better information to all stakeholders in the healthcare system.[25] It only makes sense that healthcare organizations should avail themselves of CER data where possible to optimize their operations. One may even find that the current trend of prescribing the newest medications or ordering the newest lab or imaging studies in addition to not being more effective, may expose patients to higher risks.[24] This may result in *higher* costs and *lower* quality.

FEEDBACK CONTROL OF PERFORMANCE

In the traditional model of business management, strategy was devoted to development of plans that over time would give the business advantages that would directly or indirectly result in improved financial performance. In such an environment, a quality-enhancing intervention would be treated as a project that would be adopted or turned down based on an expected rate of return on investment; unless, of course, such an intervention is mandated by a regulatory body.

With the integration of quality of care into pervasive performance metrics, in a manner similar to financial performance, the perspective of management would change in favor of analysis of every strategic and tactical decision in terms of its impact on the organization's financial *and* quality performance. With an optimal design of a quality performance measurement system customized to the needs of the healthcare organization, quality improvements can be linked and translated to financial measures and outcomes. Ideally, executives can make decisions based on conditions in the environment and priorities of the organization in a manner that is consistent with the organization's values and mission.

But the usefulness of a performance measurement system that integrates finance and quality is not limited to strategic planning. Indeed, it is useful throughout the management cycle of strategy development and execution. By intermittent status and performance assessment during execution of strategy, management can respond to changing conditions and make course corrections as often as needed. This puts even further emphasis on the significance of properly designed quality measures that can be quickly and frequently assessed and have a clear link to the mechanisms for implementation of corrective action.

A closed-loop management system can successfully link strategy and operations in an organization[26] (**Figure 9-4**).

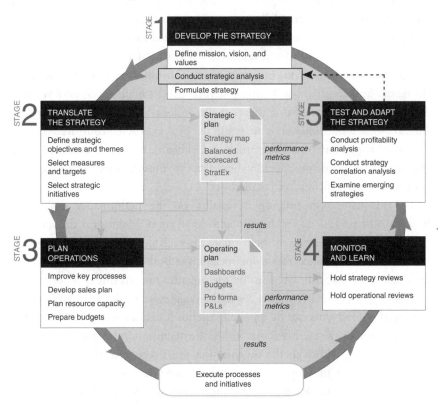

FIGURE 9-4. Closed-loop management system.[26]

Performance Dashboard

Monitoring of performance would allow management to implement course corrections hopefully in time to avoid undesirable consequences. But what does this mean in practical terms?

The answer is complex, and each organization has to design its own custom dashboard. Models such as the balanced scorecard are helpful in assessing what needs to be included. A performance dashboard must not be limited to only financial performance indicators. The nonfinancial indicators that do make it to a dashboard at the top management and governance levels have a direct impact on the cash flow of the organization either through regulatory forces or reimbursement policies such as The Joint Commission (TJC) core measures compliance and readmission rates. This raises the important point that unless there is a business case for quality, movement in the direction of quality improvement is impeded by various obstacles.[27] As important as TJC's core measures are in terms of regulatory requirements and reimbursements, they do not fully represent the quality of care delivered in an organization.

Some other nonfinancial performance indicators include customer satisfaction, market share, and human resources.[5] It is true that finance is the *lifeline* metric for the organization, but in the long run other metrics and indicators do matter and can be identified as potential drivers of financial performance. Although it is recognized that there are dimensions to performance other than finance, what these dimensions are is still the subject of some controversy.[28]

To include quality on the performance dashboard, it must be measured along the six aims of quality proposed by the IOM: care must be safe, effective, patient centered, timely, efficient, and equitable.[29]

For adequate representation of quality on the performance dashboard, healthcare organizations will have to address all six IOM aims for the care they provide. Data representing the performance in each aim will reflect the weighted averages of performance scores for specific medical diagnoses that constitute the majority of patients cared for by the organization. As discussed previously in this text, a top metric that is a weighted aggregate of the six metrics representing the IOM aims can be especially useful. It can, in one numerical value, indicate whether the quality status within the organization is steady, improving, or deteriorating, although the organization must recognize that an aggregate measure can mask underlying variation that must be corrected. This top metric is useful for internal use within the organization; however, it should not be used as a comparison tool between organizations. In addition to the six aims, other indicators representing hospital-acquired infections, medical errors, and other process indicators are essential. Finally, a breakdown of variance of the care provided in terms of overuse, underuse, and misuse will be valuable in identifying the sources of variance.[27]

REFERENCES

1. Donabedian A. Evaluating the quality of medical care. 1966. *Milbank Q.* 2005; 83(4):691–729.
2. Covey SR. *The Seven Habits of Highly Effective People.* 1st ed. New York, NY: Simon & Schuster; 1989.
3. Domain framework and inclusion criteria. Agency for Healthcare Research and Quality website. http://www.qualitymeasures.ahrq.gov/about/domain-definitions .aspx. Published 2011. Accessed November 5, 2011.
4. Carson KD, Carson PP. Strategic options for hospitals. *Hosp Top.* 1994;72(3):21.
5. Eccles RG. The performance measurement manifesto. *Harvard Business Review.* 1991; 69(1):131–137.
6. Wheeler JRC, White B, Rauscher S, et al. Pay-for-performance as a method to establish the business case for quality. *J Health Care Finance.* 2007;33(4):17–30.
7. Petersen LA, Woodard LD, Urech T, Daw C, Sookanan S. Does pay-for-performance improve the quality of health care? *Ann Intern Med.* 2006;145(4):265–272.
8. Glickman SW, Ou FS, DeLong ER, et al. Pay for performance, quality of care, and outcomes in acute myocardial infarction. *JAMA.* 2007;297(21):2373–2380.
9. Fonarow GC, Peterson ED. Heart failure performance measures and outcomes: real or illusory gains. *JAMA.* Aug 19 2009;302(7):792–794.
10. Jha AK, Joynt KE, Orav EJ, Epstein AM. The long-term effect of premier pay for performance on patient outcomes. *N Engl J Med.* Apr 26 2012;366(17):1606–1615.
11. Leatherman S, Berwick D, Iles D, et al. The business case for quality: case studies and an analysis. *Health Aff (Millwood).* 2003;22(2):17–30.
12. Snyder L, Neubauer RL, for the American College of Physicians Ethics Panel, Human Rights Committee. Pay-for-performance principles that promote patient-centered care: an ethics manifesto. *Ann Intern Med.* 2007;147(11):792–794.
13. P4P and quality care. *Trustee.* 2006; 59(7):5.
14. Ferman JH. Value-Based Purchasing Program. Part II. Payments will be based on performance. *Healthc Exec.* Jul-Aug 2011;26(4):64, 66.
15. Biffl WL, Beno M, Goodman P, et al. "Leaning" the process of venous thromboembolism prophylaxis. *Jt Comm J Qual Patient Saf.* 2011;37(3):99–109.
16. Drummond MF. *Methods for the Economic Evaluation of Health Care Programmes.* Oxford, UK: Oxford University Press; 2006.
17. Byrns RT, Stone GW. *Microeconomics.* New York, NY: HarperCollins College Publishers; 1995.
18. Committee on Redesigning Health Insurance Performance Measures, Payment, Performance Improvement Programs. P. *Medicare's Quality Improvement Organization Program: Maximizing Potential.* Washington, DC: Institute of Medicine; 2006.
19. American Recovery and Reinvestment Act of 2009. The First Session. ed 2009.
20. HHS. HHS names federal coordinating council for comparative effectiveness research. HHS website. http://www.hhs.gov/news/press/2009pres/03/20090319a .html. Published 2009. Accessed November 8, 2011.

21. Panel on effectiveness research up and running. Paper presented at: National Intelligence Report. Betheseda, MD: Institute of Management & Administration; April 13, 2009; 9:5–6.

22. J S. Researching 'comparative effectiveness' of treatments. *Workforce Management.* 2009; 88(4):26–26.

23. Laugesen MJ. Siren song: physicians, congress, and medicare fees. *J Health Politics, Policy & Law.* 2009;34(2):157–179.

24. Begley S. Why doctors hate science. *Newsweek.* 2009;153(10):49.

25. Institute of Medicine, Committee on Comparative Effectiveness Research Prioritization. *Initial National Priorities for Comparative Effectiveness Research.* Washington, DC: Institute of Medicine of the National Academies; 2009.

26. Kaplan RS, Norton DP. Mastering the management system. *Harvard Business Review.* 2008;86(1):62–77.

27. Feazell GL, Marren JP. The quality-value proposition in health care. *J Health Care Finance.* 2003;30(2):1–29.

28. Franco-Santos M, Kennerley M, Micheli P, et al. Towards a definition of a business performance measurement system. *International Journal of Operations and Production Management.* 2007;27(8):784–801.

29. Committee on Quality of Health Care in America. *Crossing the Quality Chasm: A New Health System for the 21st Century.* Washington, DC: Institute of Medicine; 2001.

CHAPTER 10

Case Studies in Healthcare Quality

INTRODUCTION

This chapter provides readers with examples of quality improvement projects that have been undertaken by healthcare organizations. The three organizations that are represented in this chapter include the Cleveland Clinic Health System, Memorial Hermann Healthcare System, and University of Southern California. These examples are not intended as a means of comparison among these institutions; indeed, all of these organizations share many similar efforts in common areas of focus in quality improvement. However, the case studies presented here illustrate that quality is a broader concept than just the reportable measures. Organizations should look beyond the regulatory requirements, as these will prove to be moving targets given the increasing and changing requirements, and focus on developing an infrastructure that allows for assessment and improvement of quality performance.

Cleveland Clinic Health System (CCHS)

In the following paragraphs, seven case studies from CCHS are presented. These case studies span a wide range of activities related to institutional strategy and infrastructure with respect to quality of care, quality improvement projects, as well as quality dashboards at CCHS. Various quality improvement toolkits and analysis methods are employed and results are discussed.

Case Study CCHS-1

How Cleveland Clinic Manages Quality of Care

Strategic Goals and Quality Management Infrastructure

J. Michael Henderson, MBChB, FRCS

The executive management team and the board of directors at Cleveland Clinic Health System (CCHS) recognized in 2006 the growing importance of implementation of a quality and safety infrastructure. They also realized that despite being a top-tier hospital system, CCHS was vulnerable to the same quality and safety problems that were plaguing health care across the country. In its assessment, leadership also recognized the need to accommodate the increasing demand for monitoring and reporting of healthcare quality data.

As a first step to remedy the situation, the goal of creating a dedicated quality infrastructure across CCHS was undertaken. This entailed consolidation and adequate resourcing of departments of quality, accreditation, clinical risk safety, infection prevention, environmental health and safety, and performance improvement. These departments, with more than 100 employees, came together in the Quality and Patient Safety Institute (QPSI), with all reporting to the chief quality officer, who in turn reports to the chief of staff. Over the subsequent 5 years, CCHS as an enterprise of 10 hospitals in Ohio and other remote healthcare locations has progressively evolved a quality and safety infrastructure. This has been based on standardization of local management with quality directors (nonphysician) and physician champions with committed time for quality and safety, leading teams that also include nursing and administrative managers in each hospital or clinical institute. The content experts from the departments in QPSI support the local teams in execution of quality goals, compliance, and performance improvement. This structure allows for decentralized ownership of quality and safety at clinical locations with umbrella oversight from enterprise-level content experts. All employees own quality and safety, and quality improvement can only be achieved at the local level.

The table of organization for quality and safety at CCHS has been changing as the above evolution has occurred to provide oversight of the CCHS program at 12 locations with more than 40,000 employees (**Figure 10-1**).

The chief quality officer, who has direct oversight of the departments in QPSI, works in close collaboration with the main campus and regional hospital quality officers who have oversight of the implementation of quality and safety in the institutes and hospitals, respectively. Strategy, goals, projects, data

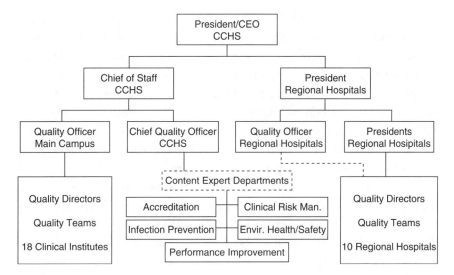

FIGURE 10-1. The organizational chart in 2012. CEO: Chief Executive Officer.

review, and accountability reside with this leadership team, which reports to executive management and the board of directors.

The senior leadership of CCHS from the hospitals and institutes participated in the strategic planning process in 2009. This consensus process is directed through the Strategic Council to the CCHS Executive Team and Directors. The quality leadership is represented in this process. CCHS's strategic clinical quality goal is to move the publicly reported quality metrics to the top decile nationally through (1) integrated infrastructure as described earlier, (2) continuous quality improvement, and (3) optimal use of data. The continuous improvement model at CCHS creates a culture of quality through a cycle of setting goals, measuring performance, improving performance, and rewarding and recognizing achievements. Improvement in quality and performance is executed through a process of define, plan, implement, and transition, using a mixed toolbox of Lean, Six Sigma, plan–do–study–act (PDSA), and FasTrac™* paradigms, among others. Use of data and performance improvement are local activities that in aggregate contribute to achievement of enterprise goals.

---

* FasTrac™ is a collaborative problem solving methodology designed by Orion Advisory, LLC (www.orionadvisory.com). The process is designed to empower teams and eliminate performance gaps, and is based on GE's WorkOut process.

Approval and funding of all CCHS initiatives and projects, both strategic and capital, follow a standard process. They are independently reviewed and scored in several areas (strategic, quality and safety, financial, growth, etc.) by six to eight members of the planning committee. The chief quality officer sits on this committee. Scores are reviewed and finalized by the committee to set funding and implementation priorities. Quality and safety receive heavy weighting in the ranking process because clinical quality is one of CCHS's top strategic priorities.

The CCHS quality dashboard is not structured according to the domains of care or the dimensions of quality as defined by the Institute of Medicine (IOM) but reports metrics in the domains of safety, quality, and patient experience. The metrics in these domains focus on reduction of harm and improvement of quality and experience outcomes in line with public reported metrics. The Cleveland Clinic board of directors (BOD) meets quarterly with active quality committees at an enterprise level and at regional hospitals. These committees meet for 1½ hours, set goals, review data, and combine this with education of the board. They report to the executive committee of the BOD. In addition, an annual retreat of the combined boards commits one-quarter to one-third of its agenda to quality and safety.

Case Study CCHS-2

Venous Thromboembolism Prophylaxis Project

Guido Bergomi

Background

Venous thromboembolism (VTE) is a major preventable cause of hospital mortality and morbidity and is also associated with significant economic burden on the healthcare system. One of the most common reasons for failure to provide appropriate VTE prophylaxis is delayed or lack of VTE risk assessment for the patients on admission.

Methods, Resources, and Performance Targets

VTE risk assessment within 24 hours of admission in adult hospitalized patients is a critical step to identify and ultimately to provide prophylaxis to patients effectively. The goal of this project was to create a uniform process to conduct the risk assessment and provide a means to measure the degree to which patients are receiving the risk assessment. The ultimate goal is to reduce the incidence of VTE.

A multidisciplinary team of physicians, pharmacists, and nurses was tasked with this project. This team investigated the full scope of the problem by examining the structure, process, and outcome domains of care. Ultimately, the team proposed a solution that required modification of the electronic health records (EHRs) system and the computerized physician order entry (CPOE) interface. Collaborating with the information technology (IT) department, the necessary programming was planned and implemented (change in structure) to put the new workflow into action (change in process). The CPOE interface was modified to require a VTE risk assessment during the admission process before admission orders could be entered. This was enhanced with best practices and decision support features and was linked to standardized evidence-based pharmacologic and non-pharmacologic VTE prophylaxis orders when indicated. A comprehensive education campaign was initiated to inform the clinicians of the project and the upcoming changes in the workflow. The education campaign included a web-based training module on the intranet as well as staff meeting presentations within various departments, physician conferences, and an announcement.

Results

The solution through the EHR requires providers to conduct the risk assessment during the admission process. By this measure, compliance is at 100% (**Figure 10-2**). Current and future efforts are centered on effective delivery of

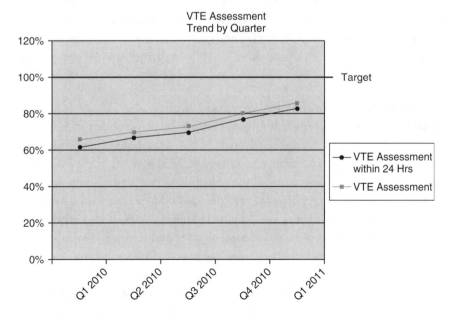

FIGURE 10-2. The process improvement results.

identified prophylaxis needs and ultimately linking these efforts to VTE outcome measures.

Conclusion

This project demonstrates use of the EHR and the CPOE interface to provide decision support, require assessment for a quality-of-care measure, require appropriate standardized and evidence-based action, and capture process measures in real time. These changes in structure and process increase efficiency, optimize allocation of resources, and reduce practice variability. The project also provided a crucial foundation to improvement of efficacy of prophylaxis and, ultimately, driving of outcomes.

This project affects three of the IOM quality-of-care aims: safety, efficiency, and patient centeredness.

Case Study CCHS-3

Surgical Site Infection Prevention Project

Guido Bergomi

Background

Surgical site infections (SSIs) are a major cause of potentially preventable patient morbidity and mortality and adversely affect healthcare costs. The incidence of colorectal infections is high and variable. A review of colorectal infections at the main campus hospital of CCHS revealed substantial opportunity for improvement.

Methods, Resources, and Performance Targets

Because of the complex, multifactorial nature of the problem, a Six Sigma DMAIC process approach was selected. In the *define* phase, the project was defined to encompass all colorectal surgery (CORS) patients at the main campus of CCHS, excluding trauma, transplant, and pediatrics subgroups, and would follow patients for 30 days postoperatively. An existing data set through the American College of Surgeons National Surgical Quality Improvement Project (NSQIP) was used to establish baseline rates and to provide measurement of ongoing progress. Stakeholders were identified to include nursing, surgeons, and quality leadership.

In the *measure* and *analyze* phases, detailed analysis was conducted using the NSQIP data set. A Pareto analysis revealed that the majority of infections were either superficial or very deep in nature. Trend charts showed a relatively stable rate of infection at about 16%. Data were analyzed using various models of cause–effect, impact–effort, benchmarking, and multivariate statistical methods. A multidisciplinary team was engaged during this time to create process maps of the preoperative, intraoperative, and postoperative processes. Process elements with potential impact on SSIs were identified and rated (**Figure 10-3**).

Ultimately, a "bundle" was identified that included elements from these processes. The bundle included:

- Preoperative Hibiclens antibacterial baths and showers
- Standard skin prep by operating room (OR) scrub nurse
- Glove and sleeve change after intraoperative digital rectal exam
- Glove and instrument change for skin closure
- Saline irrigation of incision before skin closure
- Standard application of wound dressing
- Continuation of OR dressing for 48 hours
- Mepilex dressing trial
- Clean standard dressing change as needed

During the *improve* phase, the bundle elements were communicated and implemented across the CORS group. Consistency of implementation was measured using a paper bundle checklist.

Results

The project is currently in the *improve* phase. To date, the bundle elements have been in place for roughly 3 months, with data reflecting 350 cases. Disappointingly, the overall rate has not shown a decrease. Additionally, analysis was conducted to match bundle checklist data to the NSQIP results. Because of the 30-day delay, overlap between the data sets is minimal ($n = 24$), but no statistically significant decrease was observed within this subset (**Figure 10-4**).

The team remains highly engaged in the project and is considering additional interventions to impact the measures, which include:

- Oral antibiotics with mechanical bowel preps
- Daily wound probing
- Antimicrobial incise drapes
- Wound-edge protectors
- Scalpel as opposed to cautery knife for incisions
- Preoperative nutrition therapy

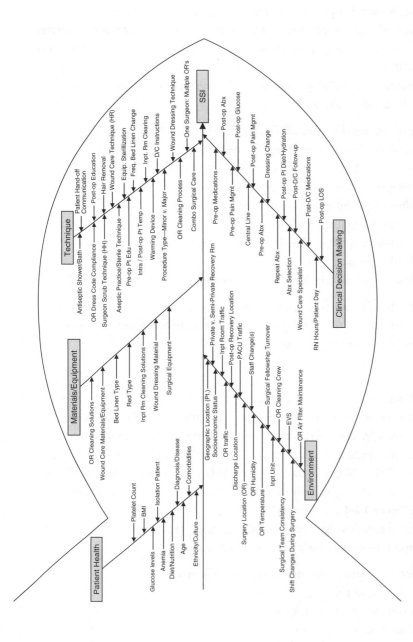

FIGURE 10-3. Detailed fishbone diagram for colorectal SSIs. OR = Operating Room, BMI = Body Mass Index, Inpt = Inpatient, RM = Room, PACU = Post-Anesthesia Care Unit, Pre-Op = Pre-Operative, Post-Op = Postoperative, Mgmt = Management, ABX = Antibiotics, RN = Registered Nurse, Equip. = Equipment, D/C = Discharge, LOS = Length of Stay, SSI = Surgical Site Infection.

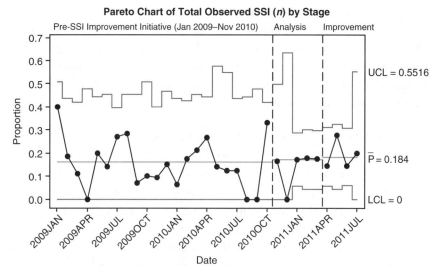

FIGURE 10-4. Colorectal SSI rates by month. UCL = Upper Control Limit, LCL = Lower Control Limit.

Conclusion

This remains an important project for CCHS. The goals of this project are aligned to the strategic quality goals of the organization, and knowledge from this team is expected to provide value across the health system. The problem of SSI is complex and tremendously multifactorial and requires an engaged team with strong leadership support to make a difference.

This project affects three of the IOM quality-of-care aims: safety, efficiency, and patient centeredness.

Case Study CCHS-4

Latex Safe Environment

Shannon Phillips, MD, MPH, Lynne Gervasi, MSN, MPA, Scott Dwyer, MBA, and John Cicero

Background

Enterprise patient safety priorities arise from many different venues—sometimes directly from the patients themselves. The CCHS chief of staff received a letter in 2007 from a parent concerned for her child. The child was highly allergic to latex and required inpatient, outpatient, and surgical care. The family could not visit CCHS facilities without constant risk of exposure to latex. There is no cure for latex allergy—avoidance of latex exposure is the only protection. Upon investigation, we discovered that latex-containing supplies were the norm in most environments. Treatment of latex-sensitive or allergic patients was considered the exception, not the rule. Often, the environmental decontamination of latex was incomplete.

Methods, Resources, and Performance Targets
For years, clinicians have assumed (and often were correct) that the quality of latex-free medical supplies and products were suboptimal compared with that of those containing latex. Our institution decided to become a latex safe (not free) environment. Latex safe seemed appropriate as not all supplies needed to care for a patient have a latex-free alternative, and several of the latex-free alternatives do not have the same quality as that of those containing latex. This project was not a financially driven initiative but rather a mission to make latex-containing supplies the exception. Creation of an environment with less exposure to latex-containing supplies would benefit patients and their families as well as our employees. Current contracts for key supplies, such as exam and surgical gloves and urinary Foley catheters, were reviewed and put out for bidding. Typically, latex-free products cost 20% to 40% more. The Executive Team supported the increased cost of latex-free gloves as it aligned with our "Patients First" approach to care. Key stakeholders to the success of this initiative included proceduralists, surgeons, nurses, urologists, supply chain staff, and ultimately our patients.

The project goals included:

- Transition all supplies used for routine patient care to a latex-free alternative if a quality alternative existed.
- Maintain quality care throughout the transition. Included were staff education and individual glove fittings.
- Set expectations around purchase of latex-free products. Negotiate favorable contracts for new products.
- Develop a mechanism to stop the ordering of latex-containing products and screen for quality latex-free equivalent products.

A multidisciplinary team was chartered to:

- Identify and label all latex-containing items in our product ordering and inventory system. Standardizing and minimizing the number of comparable products in the system would reduce clutter and gain storage.
- Conduct a cost analysis.

- Inventory and audit all storeroom items.
- Work with vendors to limit entry of latex-containing products and negotiate best prices.
- Work with clinical staff to assess the quality and fit of latex safe alternatives.
- Remove latex-free carts (previously stocked to care for latex-allergic patients) from the health system.
- Clearly mark all remaining latex-containing supplies.
- Create a patient-bedside "Latex Allergic" sign.
- Communicate the latex safe initiative through the gift shops, food service, and Cleveland Clinic physician practices so that all commercial and leased areas on our properties would adhere to the same guidelines.

Results

The initial audit revealed that of the nearly 80,000 supplies in our inventory system, approximately 1,000 contained latex. An 80/20 rule was adopted. The goal was to reach 80% latex free for our high-volume products. High-volume products included in the conversion were exam and sterile gloves and Foley and bronchial catheters. The supply chain team secured favorable contracting (**Table 10-1**). Standardizing and minimizing the number of comparable products in the system reduced confusion over selecting the right product and made it possible for the system to reduce waste and gain storage space. Most importantly, our proceduralists and surgeons were able to identify gloves that provided the necessary tactile perception and durability and catheters that met the needs of most patients in the new and improved latex-free marketplace. Several of the new latex safe products required training and follow-up education with the frontline staff. At times, the feel and flexibility of the latex-free products (catheters) was notably different (**Figure 10-5**).

Table 10-1 Cost Implications of Moving to Latex-Free Products

Supply	Volume	Cost Implication
Gloves		
Surgeon	1.4 million pairs	$1.8 million
Exam	44 million singles	Neutral
Foley catheters	40,000 units	
Silicone hydrogel		Neutral
Silicone silver alloy		$630,000
Bronchial catheters	57,000 units	$28,800 savings

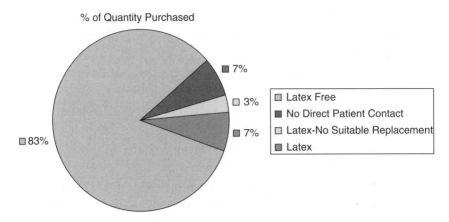

FIGURE 10-5. Distribution of supply purchases after the project.

At the conclusion of the project, the overwhelming majority of product in direct patient contact was latex free across our health system.

Conclusion

Foremost, the safety of our patients and caretakers is of singular importance. The ability to foster and deliver a culture of safety has been an ongoing mission of our health system. Addressing the risk and reality of latex allergies aligns with the health system's goals to provide the safest environment for all. Patient and employee confidence has been elevated because of the actions taken by our committee. The importance of a safety culture in creating a patient/caretaker centric, safe health care environment cannot be underestimated.

This project addressed the IOM dimensions of quality including safety and patient-centeredness.

Case Study CCHS-5

Standardization of Heparin Nomograms

Shannon Phillips, MD, MPH, and Robert Patrick, MD, MBA

Background

Cleveland Clinic identifies priorities in safety and quality through both public reporting expectations and internal monitoring and reporting systems. The internal monitoring and reporting structure for patient safety is an interdisciplinary patient safety committee led by a physician patient safety officer. This committee oversees the operation of an anonymous, voluntary intranet-based safety event reporting system (SERS), which can be easily accessed by anyone in the institution to report actual safety events or potential risks to safety. SERS entries are collated and reviewed by the committee monthly, and consistent patterns warranting further attention are identified.

Methods, Resources, and Performance Targets

Anticoagulation—thinning the blood to prevent or treat clotting—is a critical part of safe care for many hospitalized patients. The most common medication errors reported by our frontline caregivers were related to anticoagulants, specifically the intravenous anticoagulant heparin. Successful anticoagulation with heparin is measured by a blood test (PTT), which is collected 6 hours after every change in infusion rate and then daily once therapeutic levels are achieved. Heparin infusions are sometimes started with a one-time large dose of medication (bolus) in an attempt to get the patient inside the therapeutic range quickly. A PTT below the therapeutic range places the patient at risk for clotting, and above the range the risk is for spontaneous bleeding with potentially catastrophic consequences. Heparin-related SERS events were believed to be above a tolerable threshold, and consequently the patient safety committee chartered a project to improve the safety and efficacy of intravenous heparin.

Although SERS events are a good trigger for further investigation, they are anecdotal by nature and cannot accurately quantify the magnitude of any given risk. The first task of the team was to develop clinically relevant outcome measures and an information infrastructure to monitor them. Time to initial therapeutic PTT is the traditional outcome used to measure the quality of heparin therapy. This was believed to be inadequate as it measured only how fast the therapeutic range was attained and ignored what happened afterward. A new outcome was defined by the team as a percentage of time on therapy spent below/inside/above range, and initial data showed a 40%/40%/20% distribution. Detailed process mapping with key stakeholders was undertaken and showed prescribing, dosing, administration, and monitoring as the critical steps requiring intervention. Process mapping also allowed us to identify the key leads for our improvement initiative: physician staff, nursing, pharmacy, and laboratory. The team was expanded and the *plan* step of the first PDSA cycle was undertaken using a combination of Microsystems and Lean techniques. The bundle of interventions developed in this stage is detailed below:

- Ordering: physicians
  - Standardizing electronic ordering into three nomograms and limiting heparin ordering to one of the nomograms.

- Defaulting choices within the nomogram such that once a nomogram is chosen, the only remaining choice is bolus or no bolus.
- Clear visual distinction in order between bolus/no bolus.
- Order cannot be exited without choosing bolus/no bolus.
- Dosing: nurses
  - User-friendly dosing calculator similar to a smart-phone application programmed into the EMR.
  - Maximum dose limits programmed into the calculator.
  - Clear, documented nursing acknowledgment of bolus/no bolus choice from the physician order.
- Administration: nurses
  - Smart pumps synchronize with maximum dose limits in the EMR, and overdose cannot be accidentally programmed into the pump.
- Monitoring: lab and nurses
  - Decreased variation in turnaround time for PTT.
  - Visual display of an icon on a large television screen notifies the nurse that PTT is available and it is time for recalculation of dose and infusion change.

Results

Pilot sites for the intervention were chosen based on both volume of heparin use and an assessment of willingness to change. The pilot was run for 2 months with improvement from 40%/40%/20% below/inside/above range to 21%/57%/22%. Additionally, there were improvements in process measures such as the percentage of PTT lab draws completed within 15 minutes of designated time and reduction in total cycle time.

The target percentage inside range defined in the *plan* stage was a doubling from 40% to 80%, and so the *study* portion of this PDSA cycle included a detailed review of "failures" from the pilot. It revealed poor nursing documentation and continued mistakes in dosing as contributors, and consequently two additional interventions were added to the bundle:

- Dosing: nurses
  - Two nurses calculate the dose independently and check figures with each other.
- Administration: nurses
  - The same two nurses who calculated the dose together also program the pump together and record an entry in the EMR.

Conclusion

The main financial driver in previous clinical trials of anticoagulation was a decrease in cases of catastrophic bleeding associated with anticoagulation. This outcome turned out to be extraordinarily difficult to measure in a real-world setting and even more difficult to attribute directly to improved control of heparin, so there was no attempt made to calculate financial return on investment, and the project was justified solely on the merits of improvement in patient safety.

This bundle of process changes has recently been rolled out to all units in our 1,200-bed academic hospital. We continue to monitor percentage time in range and look closely for complications of treatment. Anecdotally, members of the nursing staff have increased confidence in the care they give and call out the important teamwork that has developed as a result of this improvement program.

Case Study CCHS-6

Documentation, Extraction, and Reporting Transformation Project

Shannon Phillips, MD, MPH, Kevin Anderson, MBA, Kathy Hartman, RN, MSN, and Anthony Warmuth, MPA, FACHE, CPHQ

Background

Cleveland Clinic is recognized internationally for excellent quality of care and patient outcomes, often treating those who are too sick to receive care elsewhere. Cleveland Clinic is committed to advancing quality and patient safety through continuous improvement efforts that address care delivery and outcomes in every clinical area. These efforts have identified clinical care documentation that is sparse, incomplete, and ineffective for communicating the nature and complexity of the care rendered. Generation of consistent, accurate, and complete documentation is a challenge for busy caregivers, especially as specific requirements change frequently. With the increased emphasis on value in health care, high-quality care at a reasonable cost is critical. Reimbursement and reputation are increasingly dependent on a growing list of publicly reported quality measures, most of which are derived from documentation-based abstracted and administrative claims data. As a result, accurately and efficiently documenting the care provided is a top priority.

Methods, Resources, and Performance Targets

A task force was charged with identifying, prioritizing, and operationalizing the necessary improvements to documentation tools to improve patient care, better align medical documentation with coding, and deliver improved public quality measures.

The project goal is to improve Cleveland Clinic patient care and performance on publicly reported quality measures through optimized EMR documentation and to improve clinical collaboration with the coding and revenue cycle. Correction of documentation and reporting gaps supports more effective use of resources to enhance clinical processes and achieve better real outcomes.

- No coded hospital-acquired, publicly reported condition will leave Cleveland Clinic for revenue submission until clinical accuracy is ensured.
- Each hospital-acquired condition/infection (HAC) or patient safety indicator (PSI) is an opportunity to improve clinical care and documentation.
- Clinical documentation is a critical, effective source of communication among providers, is compliant with new documentation requirements (ICD-10), and accurately reflects the quality of care delivered (as required by public measures).

This project is based on the following key values:

- Accuracy
- Consistency
- Clinical relevance
- Transparency

The project assumptions include the following:

- Require compliance with standard documentation elements that ensure an accurate and complete medical record supporting the transition to ICD-10, Meaningful Use, and quality and safety measures.
- Create simple and intuitive documentation that optimizes use of electronic health records for patients and providers.
- Place patients first and transparently document *all* relevant HACs.

Risks to the project include the following:

- Risk of underdocumentation.
- Risk of conflicting or ambiguous documentation or overdocumentation.
- Risk of documentation in the wrong place.
- Risk of noncompliant querying of providers.

The current state involves inconsistent documentation practice and limited expectations or guidance around best practice. Provider training around EHR use is function based (how-to) rather than being based on patient centeredness, clinical workflow, and optimized documentation. Currently, multiple fronts are working on documentation improvement without collaboration or coordination. There is limited collaboration between clinicians and coders to ensure effective documentation around relevant clinical conditions prior to submission for billing.

Opportunities for improvement can be found under the following:

- Documentation:
  - Standard documentation that adequately reflects the care of the patient and is complete, accurate, and discrete in format and meets the requirements of outcomes and registry reporting.
  - Expansion of education on documentation and its impact on coding and reporting of data to include residents, fellows, and attending physicians.
  - Quality measures compliance in other clinical information systems.
  - Ensure that documentation practice is well positioned for ICD-10 coding.
- Coding:
  - Make surveillance and prevalence data available to coders in real time (e.g., central line infections, hospital-acquired pressure ulcers).
  - Identify training and tools necessary for clinical documentation improvement specialists for concurrent surveillance of incomplete or conflicting documentation related to public reporting.
  - Develop a concurrent notification process to providers for clarification of ambiguous documentation.
  - Identify discrete data documentation practices that give the coder clear direction with minimal clinical oversight.
  - Develop algorithms to guide the coders/physicians with respect to quality measures—clarify when it must have medical oversight.
  - Develop institute/hospital capacity to conduct timely review of the cases that "fall out."
- Reporting:
  - Ensure the integrity of the data as it moves through numerous internal systems prior to leaving for external use (CMS, other payers, etc.).

Results

At the time of this reporting, the following deliverables have been achieved:

- Enterprise-wide participation and multidisciplinary approach to team and process.

- Inventory of best practices (nationally) with respect to medical records, its governance, abstraction, and job descriptions for clinical lead.
- Inventory of top coding issues, requirements for ICD-10 and Meaningful Use, and quality/safety metric gaps.
- Inventory of who is currently looking at our documentation (registries, reporting agencies, etc.).
- Inventory of current documentation and analysis of prior work done.
- Identification and sharing from hospitals with best practices in documentation.
- Creation of "tips" in documentation allowing institutes/hospitals to improve even in current documentation schema.
- Development of a process to real-time hold all cases coded as HAC/PSI for expedited clinical review.
- Identify and begin a high-impact project (improve documentation, improve care, improve measures).
- Strong partnerships between quality, finance, and operations through collaborations that were either loose or nonexistent prior to the program.

There has also been a 40% reduction in PSIs and HACs year after year at the CCHS main campus facility (**Figure 10-6**).

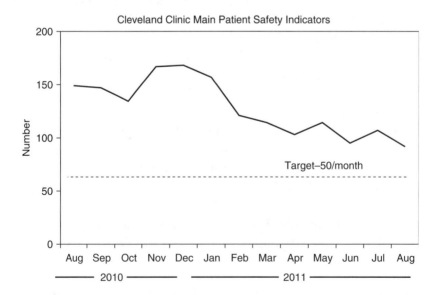

FIGURE 10-6. Patient safety indicators over time.

Conclusion

The next step in the project is the transformation to a concurrent process that allows potential HACs to be identified in real time so we can mitigate risk to patients. This provides opportunities for clinical improvement projects (several are already under way) that move beyond alignment of our documentation with the care and coding.

Case Study CCHS-7

Quality Performance Dashboards: Cleveland Clinic Health System
J. Michael Henderson, MBChB, FRCS

Data management, from collection and validation, through display and use, to accountability is challenging for all doing quality improvement. The Cleveland Clinic has invested in dashboards for all components of data that need to be shared and used across the health system. This is overseen and managed by its Enterprise Business Intelligence (EBI) team. The quality dashboard was codeveloped by the QPSI and the EBI teams and has multiple components. At the highest level, executive management has a "quality tab" on its broader dashboard, which also includes access, occupancy, finances, and other specialized areas. These dashboards are "drillable" at progressive levels for hospitals, departments, and for some metrics (such as core measures) to a physician level. In the quality arena, the dashboards are the basis for quarterly reviews by executive leadership for hospitals and departments, which is an added incentive for leaders at these levels to know their data. The same dashboards are used by the hospital boards as the data sources for board-level review of data.

A high-level view of the CCHS quality dashboard is given in **Figure 10-7**. The main component of this view is the entire health system roll-up of metrics for all hospitals in the areas of core measures, readmissions, mortality, PSIs, HACs, and hospital infections. The tabs at the top of the figure give an indication of the other domains that can be viewed and an indication of the degree to which users can drill down on the data.

Dashboards and Web tools are also used to collect and manage data in many other quality and safety scenarios. For example, CCHS has specific dashboards for ICUs, critical response teams, blood management, and others. The overall build of the dashboard allows specific locations, such as nursing floors, and functional clinical groups, such as departments, to develop specific reports relevant to their areas for tracking of progress.

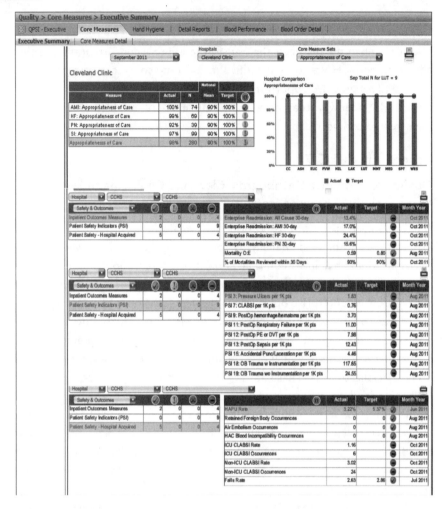

FIGURE 10-7. Screenshots of the quality dashboard at CCHS. Used by permission, Cleveland Clinic © 2012. All rights reserved.

Real-time data for quality metrics that is actionable can now be captured in some areas by either harnessing the electronic medical record, capturing events in other electronic workflows, or specifically entering data in Web tools. Examples of areas where Cleveland Clinic uses such technology are as follows:

- Assessment and ordering of VTE prophylaxis within 24 hours of hospital admission captured from a required single assessment and order form for all patients in the EMR. This feeds a "short cycle" dashboard that updates every 30 minutes and permits drill down to show which patients still have their assessment pending.

- Preoperative antibiotic timing is captured in the system-wide electronic anesthesia record. Accountability for this metric, by agreement of the perioperative team, sits with the anesthesiologist. The captured data feeds monthly staff-specific reports with patient-level detail.
- Thirty-day hospital readmissions are electronically fed to a Web tool that permits immediate feedback by department and location for all such patients with discharging and subsequent admitting physician data, diagnosis, timelines, and so forth.

Other valuable electronic tools that Cleveland Clinic and other health systems rely on in the quality and safety field are safety event reporting systems and infection prevention surveillance systems. Such systems have become essential in larger hospitals and health systems for capturing events and data, managing that data, and helping feed appropriate reporting systems. Over the next decade, standardization and simplification of such systems so that they are widely applicable in all hospitals should be a healthcare aim.

The ability to continue to develop electronic data capture that is accurate and reliably tracks performance is important, as such data capture is one of the most powerful tools available to drive standardization and reduce variability in the quality and safety field.

Memorial Hermann Healthcare System (MHHS)

Seven case studies from MHHS are presented here. These case studies encompass a wide range of topics and include a discussion of MHHS's attitude towards finance and quality as well as quality improvement projects, and quality dashboards at MHHS. As with the previous case studies, quality improvement toolkits and analysis methods are employed and results are discussed.

Case Study MHHS-1

Comparison of Finance and Quality Infrastructures at Memorial Hermann

Rachna Khatri, MPH, MBA, and William Pack, MBA

Finance and Quality: Organizational Structure Comparison

The Institute of Healthcare Improvement coined the term *the triple aim* to capture the three foci of healthcare organizations. According to Donald M. Berwick, Thomas W. Nolan, and John Whittington, "Improving the U.S. health care system requires simultaneous pursuit of three aims: improving the experience of care, improving the health of populations, and reducing per capita costs of health care."* As mentioned earlier in this chapter, hospitals have always strived for financial success and have created sophisticated and comprehensive reporting procedures to track financial performance. Recently, hospitals are being charged to work toward quality of care and also to report performance. This raises the question of how an organization's financial management processes compare to the organization's quality management processes. When comparing the financial and quality management processes at Memorial Hermann Hospital (Texas Medical Center), several similarities and differences become apparent.

Organizational Reporting Structure

Memorial Hermann has created organizational reporting structures for both quality and finance functions. **Figure 10-8** and **Figure 10-9** show the organizational charts for finance and for quality (the latter also known as the

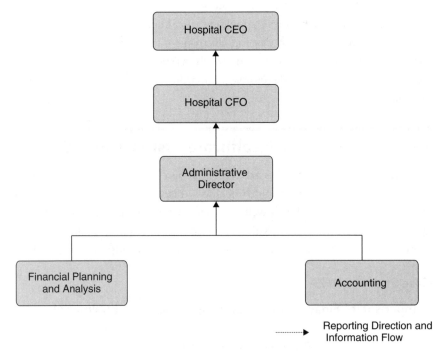

FIGURE 10-8. Memorial Hermann high-level financial reporting structure. Courtesy of Memorial Hermann Healthcare System (MHHS). CEO: Chief Executive Officer, CFO: Chief Financial Officer.

---

* Berwick DM, Nolan TW, Whittington J. The triple aim: care, health, and cost. *Health Affairs.* 2008;27(3):759–769.

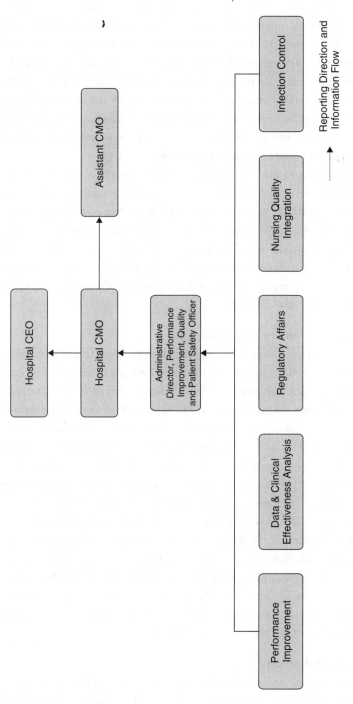

FIGURE 10-9. Memorial Hermann high-level quality reporting structure. Courtesy of Memorial Hermann Healthcare System (MHHS). CEO: Chief Executive Officer, CMO: Chief Medical Officer.

Performance Improvement and Clinical Effectiveness Department). Memorial Hermann Hospital's finance department has assigned all finance-related reporting tasks to specific individuals. A regular reporting process is in place, so that financial performance (positive and negative) can be assessed and modified in short order. By the same token, Memorial Hermann Hospital has a comprehensive quality reporting process that helps the organization track and improve processes if needed. Hospital leaders review monthly financial and quality performance reports, help set short- and long-term goals, and assist with solution formulation and administration.

This organizational design and management process is intended to begin equalizing the treatment of financial and quality performance given that financial reporting across the industry is more developed than quality reporting, and as a result, more standards exist in terms of financial performance measures and reporting methodology. Furthermore, whereas financial data is made available to all Memorial Hermann staff all the way from the C-suite to the front line, quality reporting is not as easily accessible. Quality data is typically reported to managers and senior staff.

Leadership Involvement and Incentives

Hospital leaders have always paid keen attention to financial performance, but now they are compelled to dedicate the same amount of attention to quality. First, in order for hospitals to thrive on both dimensions of finance and quality, hospital leaders must (1) be actively involved in performance assessment, and (2) support an organizational culture that empowers and encourages front-line staff to collaborate across departments and promote policies that increase revenues and improve quality. Memorial Hermann has created a structure that rallies hospital leaders to focus on six "big dots" of performance: quality and safety, patient experience, physicians, people, operational excellence, and growth. The health system has created a monthly operating report for regular performance assessment. Although the report is high level, the data can be broken down to identify performance in specific areas and departments. At Memorial Hermann, quality is given just as much emphasis as finance, as leaders' bonus payments are determined based on performance in all six "big dots." If quality performance is less than expected and financial performance is strong, executives (even the CFO) receive a lower bonus.

Information Technology

The need for accurate and timely data is essential for both finance and quality. If a patient's insurance information is not properly documented, the hospital may not receive payment for services provided. Furthermore, if a patient's blood type documented in a medical record is incorrect, the patient could suffer life-threatening consequences. As expected, effective use of IT is essential not only for financial reasons but also because it is valuable to patient care.

Hospitals have developed and improved financial reporting systems for quite some time, but the successful design and implementation of quality reporting is still a work in progress. Whereas financial reporting tends to be more auto-mated, quality reporting can often be a manual process that is time consuming and error prone. One struggle that plagues many hospitals is the integration of financial and patient care data systems, which will be necessary in the future. These challenges of bringing quality reporting up to the level of financial report-ing and of connecting the two have given rise to substantial investment in IT at Memorial Hermann.

Staff Involvement

Unfortunately, hospital physicians and staff make mistakes. Medication errors and wrong-site surgeries are just a few examples of mistakes that occur in hospitals. Medical errors reflect poor quality of care, and oftentimes the cost to repair (or mitigate the effects of) these errors are quite high. It is important for hospital staff to understand both the quality and financial consequences of provision of poor care. Patients suffer the physical and emotional effects of poor-quality care, and the payers and patients suffer increased financial burden. Just as wasting time in the OR leads to loss of revenue, so does exces-sive use of hospital supplies and equipment. Senior and junior staff must adopt a "systems" perspective to understand the close connection between quality of care and financial performance. Poor quality of care leads to poor financial performance. Of course, there is a trade-off as exceptional quality of care does not come for free, so a reasonable balance must be made to optimize care without escalating costs. As with IT, an investment in physician and staff training/education is essential in elevating quality performance management at Memorial Hermann.

Key Decision Makers: Patients

Patients choose hospitals and medical providers for various reasons. Of course, geographic proximity may dictate a patient's choice or an emergency may pre-vent time for a choice to be made. Most often, however, patients will choose a hospital based on their perception of quality of care provided at the facility. Additionally, if a patient knows that a hospital is about to go bankrupt, they may question the quality of care provided at that facility. One would expect that in the future, patient demand for quality of care *and* financial information will only increase.

When patients fail to show for a medical appointment or same-day surgery, the hospitals in general lose revenue—it is no different at Memorial Hermann. When a patient forgets to fast before an appointment and, for whatever reason, does not disclose this information to a physician, chances for poor-quality outcomes increase. Patient education that links patient behaviors to financial and quality outcomes can help boost hospital performance on both dimensions.

Closing Thoughts

The American population is very aware of the weak correlation between American's high healthcare spending and the population's health. Over the past few years, discussion of healthcare reform has opened the public's eyes to the complexity and costs of health care. As hospitals are forced to use and report more data, join shared savings plans, and work within tighter budgets, the need for closer quality and financial alignment is imminent. Diligent and reliable quality and financial reporting is important not only to internal hospital leaders but also to external stakeholders such as insurance companies, employers, healthcare workers, and patients. The truth is that hospitals today have not one but two bottom lines: finance and quality.

Case Study MHHS-2

Reduction of Turnaround Time in the Emergency Department
Yashwant Chathampally, MD, MS

Background

Emergency department (ED) overcrowding is a common problem for medical centers. Increased demand for ED services combined with increased bottlenecks in inpatient units lead to excessive delays. In this project, residents designed a system that separated care processes for level 3 patients to reduce turnaround time (TAT) and time to physician.

Methods, Resources, and Performance Targets

The aims of this project were to reduce mean TAT and mean time to physician for level 3 acuity patients by 30% within 2 months, to improve process control (i.e., reduce variation) in the target population, and to reduce the number of patients who leave without being seen (LWBS). The main process measures were total TAT and time from arrival to physician checkup for level 3 patients, and the outcome measure was the number of LWBS patients.

A Pareto chart was used to identify level 3 patients as the focus of the project, as these patients accounted for approximately 60% of total patient volume. Level 3 patients were seven times more likely than level 1 and 2 patients to be admitted (35% versus 5% admission rates). Histograms were used to identify peak times of arrival and LWBS rates. Faculty and nursing staff developed interventions in brainstorming sessions, and performance was measured with process control charts (**Figure 10-10**).

The project team set up a six-chair unit to care for level 3 patients during high-volume days and times. Level 3 patients suitable for care in the chair

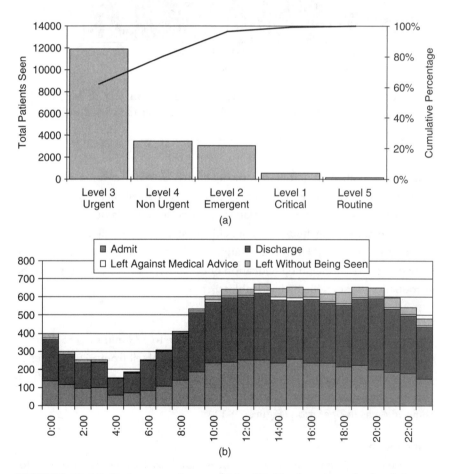

FIGURE 10-10. Preintervention analysis. (A) Total patients by level: baseline January to June 2008. (B) Emergency Center level 3: disposition by arrival time. Courtesy of Memorial Hermann Healthcare System (MHHS).

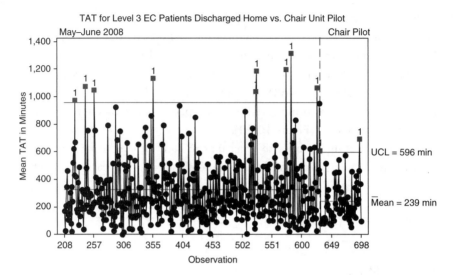

FIGURE 10-11. The results of the interventions. Courtesy of Memorial Hermann Healthcare System (MHHS). UCL: Upper Control Limits; EC: Emergency Center.

unit were classified as patients with headache, asthma, chronic obstructive pulmonary disease (COPD), extremity trauma, sickle-cell pain, low-risk chest complaints, simple urinary complaints, respiratory complaints, and eye and ENT complaints. Daily huddles were held to assess and modify care processes in the chair unit. Lastly, physical changes to the area were made to facilitate work process flow, including relocation of computers for easier access and the introduction of portable bedside tables.

Results

Mean TAT decreased from 323 minutes at baseline to 179 minutes (55% reduction), and the upper limit of the 95% confidence level fell from 970 minutes to 596 minutes, indicating reduced variation. Mean time to physician fell from 119 minutes to 64 minutes, and no patients left without being seen while the chair unit was in operation (**Figure 10-11**).

Conclusion

This project highlights the use of process analysis to identify priorities for improvement and the use of process redesign to improve patient flow. By creating a separate care process for the largest patient group, the project team was able to reduce TAT and time to physician for all ED patients. This project strengthened three of the six IOM domains of quality by improving timeliness, patient centeredness, and efficiency.

Case Study MHHS-3

Ventilator-Associated Pneumonia Reduction in a Medical ICU

Bela Patel, MD, Tammy Campos, RN, MSN, and Ruth Siska, RN

Background

Ventilator-associated pneumonia (VAP) is the leading cause of death among patients diagnosed with hospital-acquired infections. In the medical intensive care unit (MICU) at Memorial Hermann Hospital (Texas Medical Center), chief diagnoses are septicemia, respiratory failure, HIV/AIDS, renal failure, and multisystem organ failure. Roughly 60% of all patients are ventilated for more than 3 days, increasing the risk of VAP. Previous process improvement efforts reduced the MICU VAP rate from 2 to 3 per month to less than 10 per year. In this project, physicians, nurses, and process improvement professionals teamed up to develop a "bundle" of treatment plans to further reduce VAPs in the MICU to 0 within 6 months.

Methods, Resources, and Performance Targets

The key outcome measure for this project was the number of VAPs per 100 ventilator days. The main process measure was increased compliance with all aspects of the ventilator bundle. A fishbone diagram (**Figure 10-12**) was used to identify possible causes of VAP, and research uncovered preventive strategies (**Figure 10-13**) to be incorporated in the "vent bundle."

The project team designed several interventions to eliminate VAPs in the MICU. "Huddles" on VAP and mortality were held on a regular basis. VAP and compliance rates were posted in the unit for staff and physicians to see and in public areas for patients and family viewing. The project team also reviewed bundle compliance regularly in multidisciplinary team meetings and developed a physician rounding tool to address VAP bundles. Unit champions were appointed to ensure patients were out of bed, and oral care processes using chlorahexadine were formalized. Patient Care Assistants (PCAs) were trained in oral care, and the organization mandated that oral care is a shared responsibility among RNs, respiratory therapists, and PCAs. Oral care expectations were increased from 4 to 10 times per day. Computerized reminder alerts were

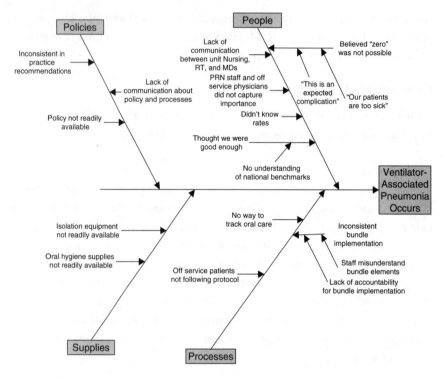

FIGURE 10-12. Preventive VAP strategies: MICU VAP fishbone diagram. Courtesy of Memorial Hermann Healthcare System (MHHS). MICU: Medical Intensive Care Unit; VAP: Ventilator Associated Pneumonia.

created for the care team, and oral care supplies were shifted closer to the ventilators. Isolation practices for all infected patients were enhanced to include booties and head coverings. Other changes included a new glycemic protocol to keep glucose between 80 and 150, an automatic insulin drip for all patients who had two consecutive finger sticks above 150, and a standardized sedation protocol. Transportation practices were reassessed and modified, and daily manager rounds were instituted to ensure bundle compliance. Infectious diseases staff worked closely with the project team by performing weekly audits and leading root-cause analysis if/when VAPs occurred.

Results

The number of VAPs fell from 8 to 12 per year to 0 within 3 months, and currently, compliance with all aspects of the VAP bundle is between 98% and

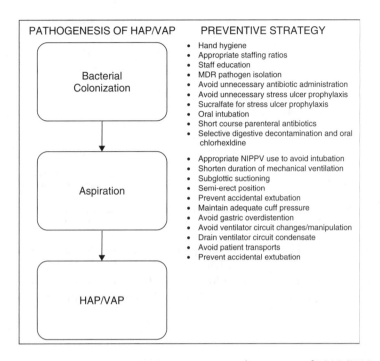

FIGURE 10-13. Preventive VAP strategies: pathogenesis of HAP/VAP and preventive strategy. HAP: Hospital Acquired-Pneumonia; MDR: Multidrug-resistant Pathogens; NIPPV: Noninvasive Positive-Pressure Ventilation; VAP: Ventilator Associated Pneumonia.
Source: Reproduced from Isakow W, Kollef MH. Preventing ventilator-associated pneumonia: an evidence-based approach of modifiable risk factors. *Semin Respir Crit Care Med.* 2006;27(1):005–017.

100%. Financial analysis indicates that a VAP adds $57,000 in additional costs for additional antibiotics, ventilator time, and ICU stay. Therefore, by preventing 8 VAPs per year, costs of $456,000 are avoided (**Figures 10-14, 10-15** and **10-16**).

Conclusion

This project shows the potential complexity of quality improvement projects and the potential quality and financial outcomes. A multipronged process improvement effort including employee training, education, and data collection and reporting resulted in a huge success by advancing four of the six IOM domains of quality: effectiveness, patient centeredness, safety, and efficiency.

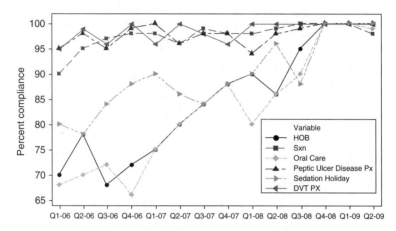

FIGURE 10-14. The results of compliance rate and VAP incidence over time: VAP bundle compliance, January 2006 to July 2009. Courtesy of Memorial Hermann Healthcare System (MHHS). HOB: Head Of Bed, Sxn: Suction, Px: Prophylaxis, DVT: Deep Venous Thrombosis.

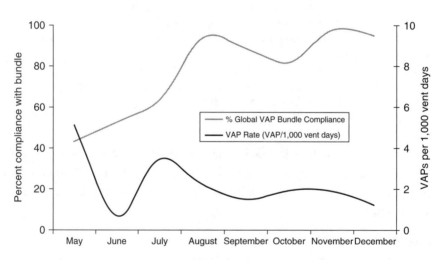

FIGURE 10-15. The results of compliance rate and VAP incidence over time. Courtesy of Memorial Hermann Healthcare System (MHHS).

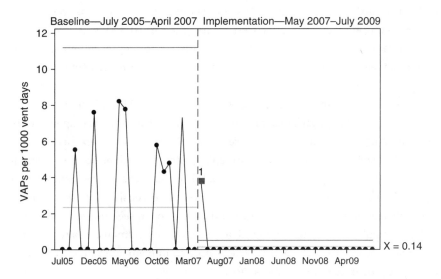

FIGURE 10-16. The results of compliance rate and VAP incidence over time. MICU-VAPs per 1,000 vent days: reduction from 2.34 to 0.14. Courtesy of Memorial Hermann Healthcare System (MHHS).

Case Study MHHS-4

Improvement of Compliance with Survival of Sepsis Goals

Bela Patel, MD, James McCarthy, MD, Tammy Campos, RN, Ruth Siska, RN, and Lillian Kao, MD, MS

Background

Sepsis is the 10th most common cause of death in the United States and the leading cause of death in the ICU. Physician, nursing, and process improvement leaders at the Memorial Hermann Hospital (Texas Medical Center) teamed up to improve sepsis resuscitation bundle (SRB) compliance and decrease mortality and length of stay (LOS) among septic patients in the MICU.

Methods, Resources, and Performance Targets

The main goal of this project was to increase mean overall compliance with the SRB within 6 hours of arrival from <5% to ≥50% within 6 months. The process measures were compliance with the individual SRB elements within 6 hours of arrival and compliance with all six SRB elements for each patient within 6 hours of arrival. The outcome measures were mortality for sepsis patients and LOS.

A fishbone diagram (**Figure 10-17**) was used to identify possible causes of noncompliance, and a process map (**Figure 10-18**) was created to understand the diagnosis and treatment process for septic patients. Pareto chart analysis helped identify bundle items that were most often incorrect (**Figure 10-19**).

The project team implemented several changes. Multidisciplinary staff, including nurses, physicians, nutritionists, and respiratory therapists, were educated on the components and use of the SRB. A sepsis screen checklist was placed in each chart for physician screening, and each unit appointed a champion to ensure education was available 24/7 in the ICU and emergency center (EC). The project team implemented standardized sepsis order sets, posted compliance rates in the unit for staff and physicians to see, and reviewed compliance regularly in team meetings. Daily rounds were administered to monitor bundle compliance in the MICU. The team also implemented mini root-cause analysis processes to review all failures.

The project team worked with other departments such as the EC and the pharmacy. Routine feedback with the EC and process redesign helped reduce transfer delays for EC patients admitted to the ICU. The Clinical Skills Center provided training on ultrasound placement education to decrease time to central line placement, and the pharmacy added drugs to Pyxis to ensure rapid access. The team also trained rapid response team nurses to incorporate sepsis screening and resuscitation outside of the ICU.

Results
Compliance with bundle elements increased from <20% in August 2006 to 60% in August 2009 (**Figures 10-20, 10-21**). Also, the MICU saw a decrease in mortality among septic patients and LOS among all risk groups (**Figures 10-22, 10-23**).

Conclusion
This is another example of how a project team achieved significant clinical quality improvement by reducing mortality among septic patients and LOS among all patients. The project highlights the importance of interdepartmental collaboration and education in achieving results. This initiative promoted five of the six IOM domains of quality: effectiveness, patient centeredness, timeliness, safety, and efficiency.

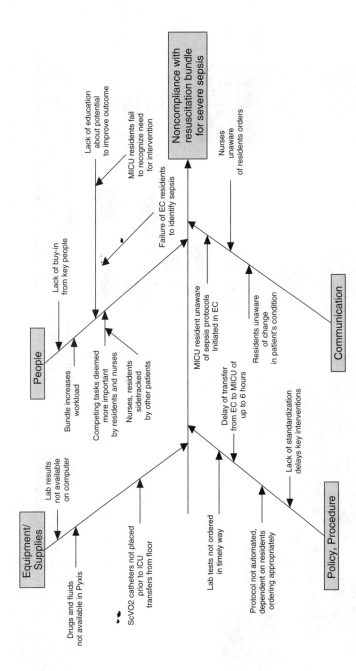

FIGURE 10-17. Preintervention analysis of the problem: bundle compliance for severe sepsis. CX: Culture; EGDT: Early Goal-Directed Therapy; MICU: Medical Intensive Unit; EC: Emergency Center; RRT: Rapid Response Team; MD: Physician; ABG: Arterial Blood Gas; AB: Antibiotics; ScVO2: Central Venous O2 Saturation. Courtesy of Memorial Hermann Healthcare System (MHHS).

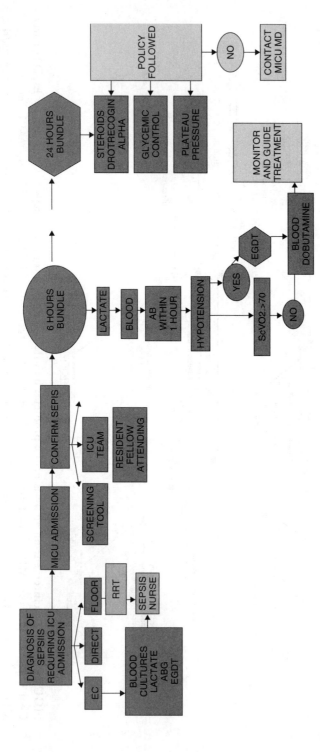

FIGURE 10-18. Pre-intervention analysis of the problem: process map. CX: Culture; EGDT: Early Goal-Directed Therapy; MICU: Medical Intensive Unit; EC: Emergency Center; RRT: Rapid Response Team; MD: Physician; ABG: Arterial Blood Gas; AB: Antibiotics; ScVO2: Central Venous O2 Saturation. Courtesy of Memorial Hermann Healthcare System (MHHS).

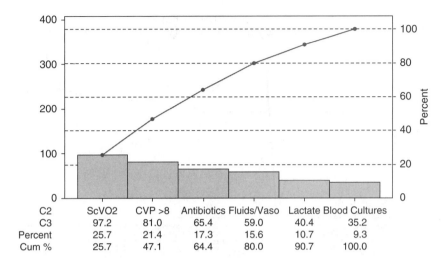

	ScVO2	CVP >8	Antibiotics	Fluids/Vaso	Lactate	Blood Cultures
C2 C3	97.2	81.0	65.4	59.0	40.4	35.2
Percent	25.7	21.4	17.3	15.6	10.7	9.3
Cum %	25.7	47.1	64.4	80.0	90.7	100.0

FIGURE 10-19. Preintervention analysis of the problem: percentage incorrect per bundle item. Courtesy of Memorial Hermann Healthcare System (MHHS). Cum: Cumulative, Vaso: Vasopressor, CVP: Central Venous Pressure, ScVO2: Central Venous O2 Saturation.

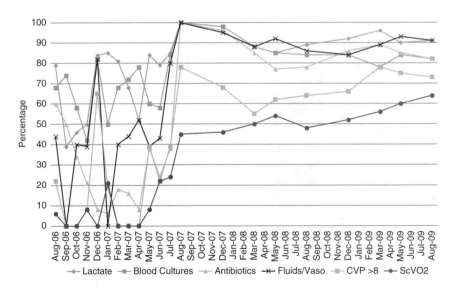

FIGURE 10-20. The results of the interventions: compliance with bundle elements. Courtesy of Memorial Hermann Healthcare System (MHHS). CVP: Central Venous Pressure, ScVO2: Central Venous O2 Saturation.

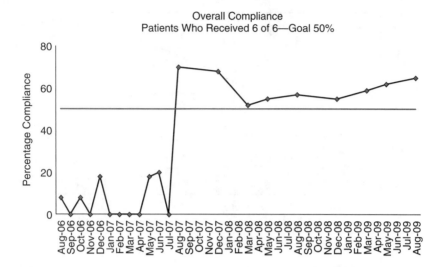

FIGURE 10-21. The results of the interventions: overall compliance. Courtesy of Memorial Hermann Healthcare System (MHHS).

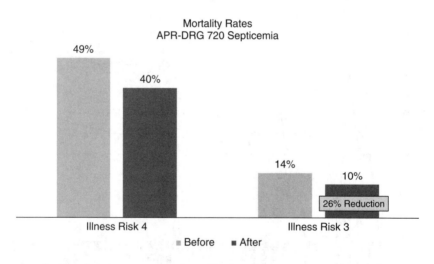

FIGURE 10-22. The results of the interventions: mortality rates. Courtesy of Memorial Hermann Healthcare System (MHHS). APR-DRG = All Patient Refined Diagnosis Related Groups.

| Length of Stay in Days | | | |
| APR-DRG Illness Risk | | | |
1-Mild	2-Moderate	3-Major	4-Extreme
Before	4.7	7.1	7.7	12.0
After	3.5	5.5	6.8	10.6
Decrease	1.2	1.5	0.9	1.4
% Decrease	25%	22%	12%	11%

FIGURE 10-23. The results of the interventions: length of stay in days. Courtesy of Memorial Hermann Healthcare System (MHHS). APR-DRG = All Patient Refined Diagnosis Related Groups.

Case Study MHHS-5

Reduction in Transfer Time from the Emergency Room to the ICU

Pratik Doshi, MD, Brent King, MD, James McCarthy, MD, Bela Patel, MD, Yashwant Chathampally, MD, MS, Ruth Siska, RN, Tammy Campos, RN, MSN, Sylvia Reimer, RN, Janice Hughes, RN, and Katharine Luther, RN, MPN

Background

Emergency department patients requiring admission to the ICU often experience substantial transfer delays. Studies have shown that delays exceeding 4 hours result in increased hospital mortality, hospital LOS, and ICU LOS.[*] The main goal of this quality improvement initiative was to reduce the transfer time for ED patients admitted to the ICU and consequently reduce hospital mortality and LOS.

Methods, Resources, and Performance Targets

Mean time from completion of ED care to arrival in the MICU was defined as the process measure, and hospital mortality for ICU patients, hospital LOS for ICU patients, and ICU LOS were defined as outcome measures.

Graphical analysis indicated that the process step with the highest variation (**Figure 10-24**) was "care complete to departure," and Pareto chart analysis (**Figure 10-25**) helped identify key reasons for delay. After observing that >50% of patient delays occurred when clean beds were available, box plots were created (**Figure 10-26**). Process maps were used to understand current processes, identify problem areas, and design solutions.

---

[*] Chalfin et al. Impact of delayed transfer of critically ill patients from the emergency department to the intensive care unit. *Crit Care Med*. 2007;35:1477–1483.

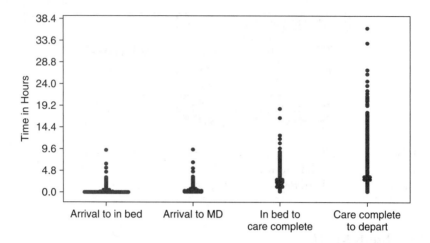

FIGURE 10-24. Preintervention analysis of the problem: MICU admits from EC. Courtesy of Memorial Hermann Healthcare System (MHHS).

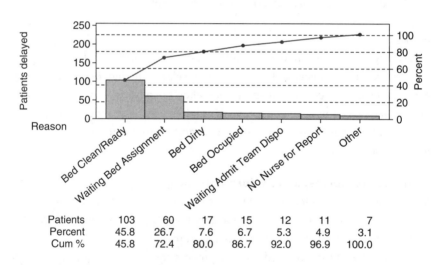

	Patients	103	60	17	15	12	11	7
	Percent	45.8	26.7	7.6	6.7	5.3	4.9	3.1
	Cum %	45.8	72.4	80.0	86.7	92.0	96.9	100.0

FIGURE 10-25. Preintervention analysis of the problem: reasons for delays in transfer to MICU, September to October 2009. Courtesy of Memorial Hermann Healthcare System (MHHS). Dispo: Disposition, Cum%: Cumulative Percentage.

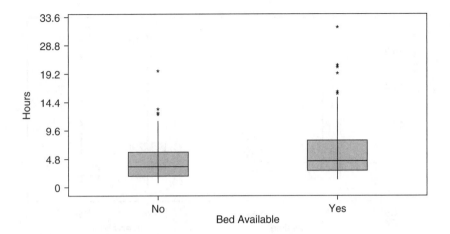

FIGURE 10-26. Preintervention analysis of the problem: boxplot of care complete to departure. Courtesy of Memorial Hermann Healthcare System (MHHS).

Several interventions were rolled out to expedite transfer time for ED patients admitted to the ICU. The project team created a qualifying admission tool and prequalifying checklist to speed along ED processes, and the team established standardized nursing documentation for recording departure time data. The team worked with ICU, ED, and bed management staff to redesign the bed request and assignment processes.

Results

The mean time from ED care complete to MICU admission decreased 37% from 5.53 hours to 3.49 hours, and the mean time for ED LOS (arrival to departure) fell 22% from 8.81 hours to 6.83 hours. The variation in the latter process decreased as the standard deviation fell from 5 hours 46 minutes to 4 hours 12 minutes. Total ED LOS for ICU patients assigned to clean/available beds fell from 9 hours 21 minutes to 2 hours 34 minutes, and total LOS for MICU patients admitted from the ED decreased from 9.67 to 8.13 days (p value of 0.0035). No change in mortality rates resulted, but according to financial analysis, the 1.54 decrease in LOS for 643 MICU admissions from the ED amounted to 990 fewer ICU days and $1,039,500 in reduced costs over the year (**Figures 10-27** and **10-28**).

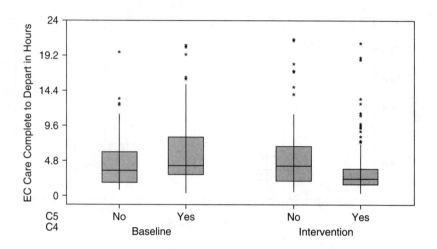

FIGURE 10-27. The results of the intervention: care complete to departure versus MICU bed availability. Courtesy of Memorial Hermann Healthcare System (MHHS). EC = Emergency Center.

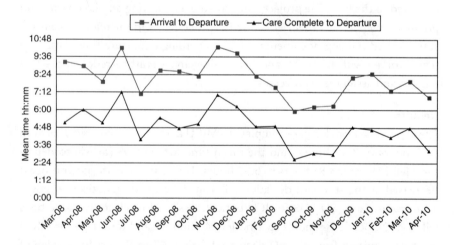

FIGURE 10-28. The results of the intervention: mean time of arrival to departure versus care complete to departure. Courtesy of Memorial Hermann Healthcare System (MHHS).

Conclusion

Several hospitals suffer from ED to ICU transfer delays. This project is yet another illustration of how improvement in process efficiency for one patient group (MICU) can improve process flow for other patients. This project advanced five of the six IOM domains of quality: effectiveness, patient centeredness, timeliness, safety, and efficiency.

Case Study MHHS-6

Serious Safety Events Classification System

M. Michael Shabot, MD, and Rachna Khatri, MPH, MBA

Documentation of serious safety events is critical to any healthcare organization, as timely reporting of serious safety events enables the organization not only to keep track of errors but also to create methods to prevent such errors from reoccurring. To better understand and react to serious safety events, the Memorial Hermann system adapted a classification system originally developed by Healthcare Performance Improvement, Inc., for its internal purposes. The classification system in general is used by several hundred hospitals nationwide and helps organizations categorize and prioritize serious safety events. Potential or actual safety events are initially classified into three groups: good catches, close call events, and serious safety events (**Figure 10-29**).

Good catches are errors or potential accidents that were caught by one of multiple safety barriers that have been created in various systems of care. At Memorial Hermann, our EHR makes upwards of a thousand good catches a month, warning and convincing physicians, nurses, and pharmacists to avoid certain medications, combinations of medications, and treatments.[*,†]

Close call events are potentially adverse events not related to the patient's illness, injury, or underlying condition that could have caused significant harm, but did not. Close call events are carefully investigated.

Serious safety events (SSEs) are actual adverse events not related to the patient's illness, injury, or underlying condition that actually did cause a degree of harm. SSEs are investigated with a root-cause analysis.

---

[*] Bates DW, Cohen M, Leape LL, Overhage JM, Shabot MM, Sheridan T. Reducing the frequency of errors in medicine using information technology. *J Am Med Inform Assoc.* 2001;8(4):299–308.

[†] Selvan MS, Sittig DF, Thomas EJ, Arnold CC, Murphy RE, Shabot MM. Improving erythropoietin-stimulating agent administration in a multihospital system through quality improvement initiatives: a pre-post comparison study. *J Patient Saf.* 2011;7(3):127–132.

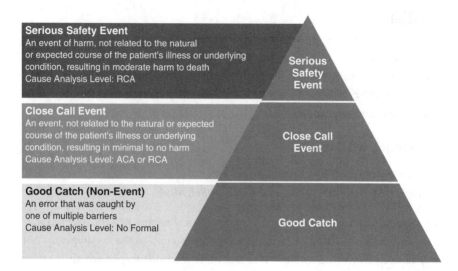

FIGURE 10-29. Serious safety event classification (Memorial Hermann Healthcare System, as modified from Healthcare Performance Improvement, Inc.). RCA: Root Cause Analysis; ACA: Apparent Cause Analysis. Courtesy of Healthcare Performance Improvement, LLC.

SAFETY EVENT CLASS	LEVEL OF HARM	CODE	DESCRIPTION
SERIOUS SAFETY EVENT	Death	SSE1	Death due to injury or error, not related to the natural or expected course of the patient's illness or underlying condition.
	Severe Permanent Harm	SSE2	Detectable harm due to injury or error, causing great discomfort, injury, and/or distress (including permanent loss of organ function), not related to the natural or expected course of the patient's illness or underlying condition.
	Moderate Permanent Harm	SSE3	Detectable harm due to injury or error, greater than minimal harm but less than severe harm (e.g., chronic renal insufficiency post acute renal failure), not related to the natural or expected course of the patient's illness or underlying condition.
	Severe Temporary Harm	SSE4	Detectable harm due to injury or error, lasting for a limited time only, resulting in no permanent injury, yet causing great discomfort, injury, and/or distress (e.g., additional procedure, surgery, or resuscitation), not related to the natural or expected course of the patient's illness or underlying condition.
	Moderate Temporary Harm	SSE5	Detectable harm due to injury or error, lasting for a limited time only, resulting in no permanent injury and is greater than minimal harm, but less than severe harm (e.g., does not require additional surgery, procedure, or resuscitation measure), not related to the natural or expected course of the patient's illness or underlying condition.
CLOSE CALL EVENT	Minimal Permanent Harm	PSE1	Detectable harm due to injury or error, not expecting change in clinical status and is minimal in severity (e.g., scar from laceration), not related to the natural or expected course of the patient's illness or underlying condition.
	Minimal Temporary Harm	PSE2	Detectable harm due to injury or error, lasting for a limited time only, resulting in no permanent injury and is minimal in severity; requires little or no intervention, not related to the natural or expected course of the patient's illness or underlying condition.
	No Detectable Harm	PSE3	Not able to discover or ascertain the existence, presence or fact of harm due to injury or error, but harm may exist; insufficient information available or unable to determine any harm
	No Harm	PSE4	The absence of harm due to injury or error, with sufficient information available to determine that no harm occurred (i.e., "got lucky").
GOOD CATCH	Event "almost happened"	NME1	Error, injury, or condition was caught by an error detection barrier (i.e., the system worked)
	Adverse-to-Quality Condition	NME2	Requires remediation but not an apparent or root cause analysis process.

FIGURE 10-30. Serious safety event classification system (Memorial Hermann Healthcare System, as modified from Healthcare Performance Improvement, Inc.). Courtesy of Healthcare Performance Improvement, LLC. NME = Near Miss Safety Event

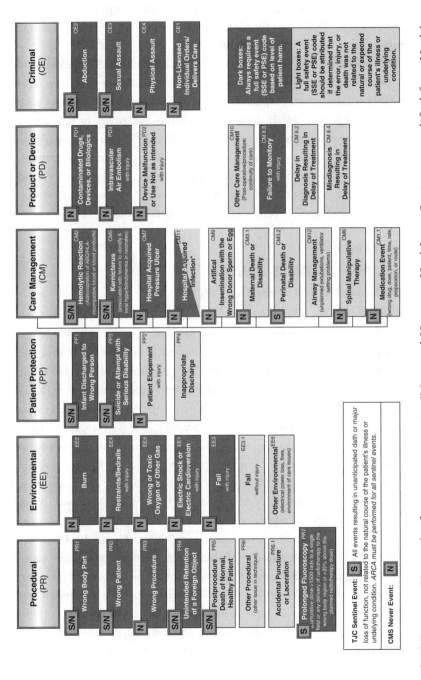

FIGURE 10-31. Hospital safety event categories (Memorial Hermann Healthcare System, as modified from Healthcare Performance Improvement, Inc.). Courtesy of Healthcare Performance Improvement, LLC.

A finer level of detail is required to classify the degree of harm associated with SSEs and close call events. That detail is provided in **Figure 10-30**, which provides five levels of SSEs and four levels of close call events. Close call events are abbreviated as "PSEs" for *potential safety events*.

In the Memorial Hermann Healthcare System, all SSEs and PSEs are reviewed monthly in a special meeting of chief medical officers, chief nursing officers, chief executive officers, and system executives. Actions plans are formed and managed to prevent similar SSEs and PSEs across the healthcare system in the future.

An even finer level of detail is provided for hospital safety event categories in **Figure 10-31**. This allows events to be classified in terms of cause: procedural, environmental, patient protection, care management, product/device, and criminal. Subitems that are classified as "sentinel events" by The Joint Commission or "never events" by CMS are marked with a special indicator.

Case Study MHHS-7

Quality Performance Dashboards

M. Michael Shabot, MD, and Rachna Khatri, MPH, MBA

Memorial Hermann Healthcare System in Houston, Texas, has created a Flash Report Dashboard to keep track of quality and safety performance metrics. The dashboard is not only an effective means of identification of problem areas but also enables the organization to track performance and determine whether an intervention was effective. Furthermore, the Flash Report Dashboard promotes department- and facility-level comparisons, which could be invaluable in recognition of areas with best practice. The flash report is available as an intranet Web application on all management computer workstations via a special icon that resides in the "system tray" at the bottom right of PC screens and that flashes when new data have been loaded. Administrative, volume, and financial data are current to midnight of the prior day. Quality and safety data are also available in real time, although monthly results are not complete until a few days after the month closes. **Figure 10-32** shows a flash report of core measure compliance for a Memorial Hermann acute care hospital. **Figure 10-33** shows a flash report of hospital-acquired infection measurements and central line safety bundle compliance for a different acute care hospital.

Additionally, Memorial Hermann has found performance dashboards to be an effective tool for process improvement. After an extensive strategic planning

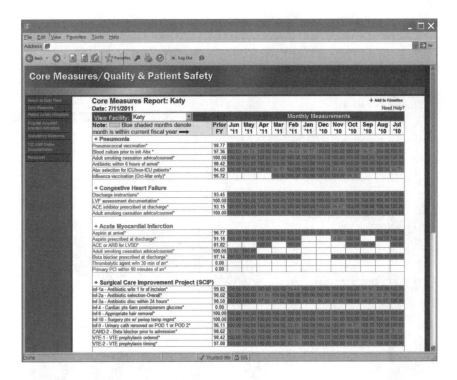

FIGURE 10-32. Core measure flash report (internal web, Memorial Hermann Healthcare System). Courtesy of Memorial Hermann Healthcare System (MHHS).

process, leaders from the adult ICUs from across the Memorial Hermann system believed they needed a comprehensive monthly report to assess the effectiveness of care in each individual ICU. A steering committee was created, and performance measurements were eventually selected from a long list. After several months of development, a totally automated process was developed to produce individual monthly ICU metrics dashboards for each of 20 adult ICUs and a summary of combined performance. The report is automatically generated in portable document format (PDF) form and e-mailed to each ICU director, nurse manager, and chief medical officer (**Figure 10-34**). Each person receives a complete report for all 20 ICUs and the summary, which provides total transparency for ICU performance across the health care system. Performance in almost all areas has improved since the report went into production

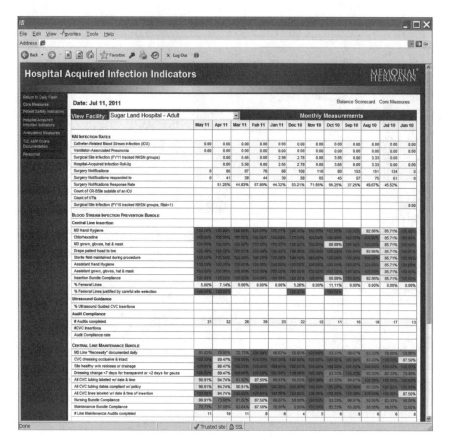

FIGURE 10-33. Hospital-acquired infection and bundle compliance flash report (internal web, Memorial Hermann Healthcare System). Courtesy of Memorial Hermann Healthcare System (MHHS).

several years ago. Comparative results are discussed at ICU director and nurse manager meetings throughout the year.

Figure 10-35 shows a highly summarized dashboard for quality, safety, patient experience, physician satisfaction, employee satisfaction and retention, and financial and growth performance measures developed at the Memorial Hermann Healthcare System.

Unit Abbreviation	HH-ICU Medical ICU
Unit Name	TMC-MICU (MICU)
Medical Director	Bela Patel, MD
Nursing Director	Ruth Siska, Carmelita McKnight, Allison Harse, RN's

	April	March	February	6 Month Avg	12 Month Avg	Current vs. 12-mo Trend	Notes
Operating Beds	16.0	16.0	16.0	16.0	16.0	No Change (<1%)	
Discharges	128.0	135.0	127.0	128.0	127.2	No Change (<1%)	
Occupancy	92.1%	89.1%	91.4%	89.6%	86.5%	Increase of 6.4%	
Average ICU Length of Stay (days)	3.45	3.27	3.22	3.38	3.31	Increase of 4.3%	
Average Hospital Length of Stay (days)	11.95	12.79	15.43	11.93	11.39	Increase of 4.9%	
% IMU/Routine Room Charges	6.7%	8.0%	7.8%	7.6%	7.4%	Decrease of 9.9%	
ICU Glucose Monitoring							
Bedside glucose measurements per day	5.99	6.87	7.62	6.37	7.08	Decrease of 15.5%	All measurements
Hypoglycemia <60 mg/dL	0.4%	0.3%	1.3%			Decrease of 49.1%	Excludes first 24 hrs
Hyperglycemia >200 mg/dL	3.4%	7.3%	N/A	N/A	N/A		Excludes first 24 hrs
ICU HAI Bundle Compliance							
VAP Bundle Compliance - MD			93.2%	94.7%	90.2%	Decrease of 7.8%	Average of system ICUs
VAP Bundle Compliance - Nursing					94.3%	Increase of 3.5%	Average of system ICUs
CR-BSI Insertion Bundle Compliance	100.0%		88.9%			Increase of 2.7%	Average of system ICUs
CR-BSI Line Maintenance Compliance	92.9%	88.9%	91.7%	85.5%	87.4%	Increase of 6.3%	Average of system ICUs
ICU Utilization							
Epotin cost per ICU day	$0.00	$0.25	$0.14	$0.61	$1.00	Decrease of 100%	Procrit & Aranesp for non-ESRD
Nicardipine cost per ICU day	$6.93	$2.66	$8.47	$6.59	$8.14	Decrease of 14.9%	Cardene only
Propofol cost per ventilator day	$0.88	$1.29	$1.21	$1.02	$1.34	Decrease of 34.6%	
Antibiotics cost per day	$115.04	$116.51	$124.22	$91.08	$80.57	Increase of 42.8%	
Average # Ventilator Days			4.61			Increase of 2%	For ventilated patients only
Vent-to-Trach Days	9.67	8.50	8.00	6.57	6.68	Increase of 44.7%	Excludes same-day trachs
% Avoidable ICU Days		0.9%	1.0%	3.5%	4.2%	Decrease of 29.9%	*Subject to reporting*
ICU Costs & Margin							
Total Indirect cost per patient day	$1,142	$1,253	$1,205	$1,170	$1,175	Decrease of 2.8%	
Total Direct cost per Patient day	$2,697	$3,025	$2,824	$2,723	$2,756	Decrease of 2.1%	
Laboratory	$375	$387	$389	$378	$395	Decrease of 4.9%	
Chargeable Supplies	$425	$452	$456	$449	$451	Decrease of 5.9%	
Pharmacy	$374	$623	$492	$410	$413	Decrease of 9.5%	
Radiology	$105	$111	$102	$102	$104	Increase of 1.5%	
Respiratory	$144	$109	$93	$107	$111	Increase of 29%	
Room & Other	$1,274	$1,342	$1,292	$1,278	$1,282	No Change (<1%)	
Contribution Margin per ICU Case[1]	$7,956	$13,858	$1,558	$7,382	$6,885	Increase of 15.6%	
ICU Outcomes							
% Readmissions	11.3%	7.5%	5.4%	6.4%	8.3%	Increase of 36.7%	
Within 48 hrs leaving ICU						Increase of 97.8%	
After 48 hrs leaving ICU	4.0%	3.7%	0.8%	2.9%	4.6%	Decrease of 12.1%	
% Mortality	7.8%	6.3%	6.3%	7.7%		Decrease of 6.1%	
High Risk[a] (APR-DRG)	Delayed 1 month			7.5%			APR-DRG ROM = 3 or 4
Low Risk[a] (APR-DRG)	Delayed 1 Month						APR-DRG ROM = 1 or 2

FIGURE 10-34. Monthly ICU metrics dashboard (Memorial Hermann Healthcare System). Courtesy of Memorial Hermann Healthcare System (MHHS).

FIGURE 10-35. Board of directors dashboard. Note: Certain measures have been redacted. Courtesy of Memorial Hermann Healthcare System (MHHS).

University of Southern California (USC)

This chapter will end with presenting two case studies from USC. These case studies highlight the similarities and difference between organizations and their approach to common challenges in their quest for quality improvement. Quality improvement toolkits and analysis methods are employed and results are discussed.

Case Study USC-1

Safe Medication Administration: Interruption-Free Zones

Kathy Coe, RN, BSN, and Daniel Hudson, RN, BSN

Background

Medication administration is one of the most frequent activities performed by health care professionals while patients are admitted in a hospital.[*] Recently, media attention on medication errors has begun to bring to the fore the importance of safe medication administration practice by health care professionals, and as we move into the future of health care, this process will continue to be one of the most important tasks performed. Approximately 18.7% of all interruptions of a registered nurse per day arise when nurses are preparing or administering medications.[†] Interruptions cause a stop in the process of administering medications directly leading to medication errors, which calculate to an annual estimated adverse drug event cost of $3.5 billion.[‡] In this project, nursing leadership, focusing on patient safety, created a Medication Administration Safety Team composed of nursing management, charge nurses, direct bedside nurses, and nurse educators to innovate a concept that has already proved to be effective in decreasing interruptions to health care professionals administering medications in many other hospitals throughout the United States. Out of this team the Interruption-Free Zone Medication Administration process was created using an interruption-free zone neon yellow sash, and interruptions during medication administration were decreased from 77% to <40% within 1 month.

---

[*] McGillis Hall L, Pedersen C, Fairley L. Losing the moment: understanding interruptions to nurses' work. *J Nurs Adm*. 2010;40(4):169–176.

[†] Biron AD, Lavoie-Tremblay M, Loiselle CG. Characteristics of work interruptions during medication administration. *J Nurs Scholarsh*. 2009;41(4):330–336.

[‡] Aspden P, Institute of Medicine Committee on I, Preventing Medication E. *Preventing Medication Errors*. Washington, DC: National Academies Press; 2007.

Methods, Resources, and Performance Targets

The core outcome measure for this process improvement was interruptions during the medication administration process, and the goal was to decrease significantly the total amount of interruptions by all health care professionals to the registered nurse per medication administration. Through root cause analysis, we determined that interruptions during a section of the medication administration process directly led to a medication error; therefore, we began to research literature about this variable. Nursing management held phone conferences with other hospitals that had previously implemented similar processes to decrease interruptions and decided that a team needed to be established to address this problem. The core team was then developed using highly motivated employees, and meetings were held to discuss innovating the process for our hospital. The core team developed a data collection tool to measure the number of interruptions per medication administration pre-implementation and for 4 weeks after implementation. Two pilot units were identified (medical–surgical orthopedics and medical ICU), and bedside registered nurses were educated on the process through nursing operations and nursing quality meetings as a tool to recruit super-users to help collect data and ensure the process was performed correctly.

Through biweekly meetings, educational strategies were developed with the assistance of the marketing department, data collection super-users were assigned to each pilot unit for 6-hour time slots, and homework was assigned to each team member to aid in decreasing the amount of nonproductive time used for the project. Each unit was educated using a method of 1:1 review of literature, purpose of process improvement, and goals. This education was done by the super-users and the charge nurses of each pilot unit in order to have buy-in by the frontline staff. Daily "huddle" discussions also took place each shift during the implementation in the nursing units. The interruption-free zone piloted by the nurses was a neon yellow vest and sash. The units were asked to vote on which interruption-free zone they concluded was of easiest use, served the proper purpose, and could be seen from a 360-degree angle. The pilot units decided that the neon yellow sash was the most appropriate interruption-free zone, and this was manufactured for an extremely low cost per sash. The nurses don the interruption-free zone sash during each medication administration to indicate they are currently passing medications and to not interrupt them unless in an emergency.

Results

Before implementation of the process, data collection illustrated that 77% of all medication administrations performed in each unit were interrupted at some point of the process. The top three interruptions in descending order were patients, registered nurses, and doctors. Educational methods were directly aimed at these three groups, which the team believed were controlled variables. Through continued education daily and implementation of the process, the number of interruptions decreased in week 1 to 58%, week 2 to 49%, week 3 to 41% and finally in week 4 to 40%. Additionally, we found that the average time per medication administration decreased from 12 minutes to 8 minutes, which saved up to 30 minutes per shift depending on the number of medication administrations completed (**Figures 10-36** through **10-40**).

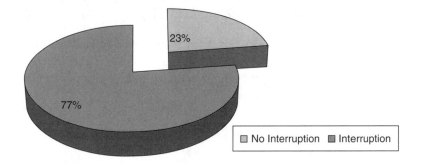

FIGURE 10-36. Results: Percentage of interruption per medication administration, preimplementation. Courtesy of Keck Medical Center of USC.

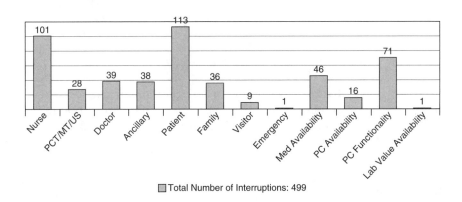

FIGURE 10-37. Results: Distribution of interruptions after implementation of the interruption-free zone, week 1. PCT: Patient Care Technician; MT: Medical Technologist; US: Unit Secretary. Courtesy of Keck Medical Center of USC.

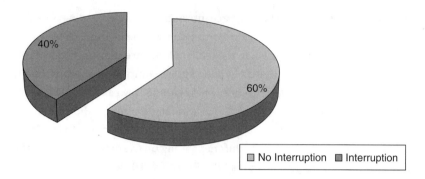

FIGURE 10-38. Results: Percentage of interruption versus no interruption per medication administration, week 4. Courtesy of Keck Medical Center of USC.

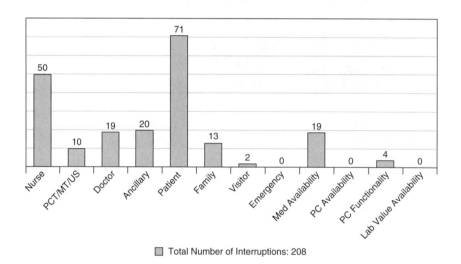

FIGURE 10-39. Results: Distribution of interruptions after implementation of the interruption-free zone, week 4. PCT: Patient Care Technician; MT: Medical Technologist; US: Unit Secretary. Courtesy of Keck Medical Center of USC.

Conclusion

This process improvement, aimed at the IOM's patient safety goal, specifically showed that nurses are interrupted a significant number of times during medication administration and that by using the interruption-free zone sash, the number of interruptions can be decreased. The data also showed that by decreasing

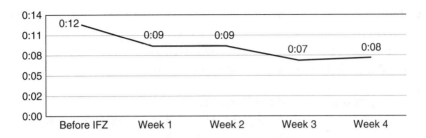

FIGURE 10-40. Results: Average time in minutes of medication administration. Courtesy of Keck Medical Center of USC. IFZ = Interruption Free Zone.

the interruptions, the nurses will have more time to be at the patient's bedside to perform other tasks and to provide education to the patients and their families, thus focusing on patient centeredness. One of the most intriguing quotes by one of the registered nurses during the pilot study was "when I place on the yellow sash it allows me to concentrate easier." Allowing our health care professionals to concentrate without interruption during medication administration is our number one goal to reduce and eliminate medication errors. This process is a step in that direction.

Case Study USC-2

Creation of a Culture of Collective Responsibility and Accountability to Patient Care Using an Interdisciplinary Approach to Improve Hospital-Acquired Infections

Kamyar Afshar, DO, and Yin Tchen RN, MHA, JD

Background
The 7 South Intensive Care Unit is a designated 18-bed neurosciences ICU at the Keck Hospital of USC. However, the unit also serves pulmonary critical care patients, postsurgical otolaryngology and orthopedic patients, and any other potential overflow patients requiring intensive care. The challenges facing 7 South ICU included a high turnover in the daily volume of patients (up to 23 patient contacts), high bedside RN administrative responsibilities, and high utilization of registry nurses due to low RN retention rates. Although the patients were receiving adequate care, there was a less than ideal and consistent communication with patients and families on the current status and/or direction of care and with participating disciplines or departments,

such as quality control, nursing infection control, respiratory therapy, and pharmacy.

In this case study, we will focus on the strategies implemented to improve hospital-acquired infections in our ICU using an interdisciplinary model.

Method, Resources, and Performance Targets

After a root-cause analysis study was completed regarding hospital-associated infections, an interdisciplinary approach was implemented consisting of a physician champion and nursing leaders collaborating with all ancillary departments to conduct daily interdisciplinary rounds focused on reducing hospital-acquired infections such as CLABSI, catheter-acquired urinary tract infection (CAUTI), and VAP with the goals of reducing morbidity, mortality, and healthcare costs. The primary goals were to improve quality, efficiency, and patient-focused care. Additional goals included increasing the availability and access to various disciplines and reducing the administrative burden on bedside nurses in order to increase focus on direct patient care. The team implemented an active surveillance tool to integrate quality of care and safety measures during the daily rounds. It monitored skin care, the number, location, and continued need of central lines and Foley catheters, and compliance with core bundle measures and safety measures (e.g., room setup/emergency equipment). This tool allowed the team to foster a proactive approach to all ICU measures in the healthcare delivery for the patients. All healthcare providers would communicate and share complete and unbiased information regarding the patient. Bedside teaching would inform and empower all team members concerning disease processes and goals for the day.

Results

There were tangible results obtained as evidenced by decreased use of central venous catheters and Foley catheters. The primary goals were obtained with the elimination of CLABSI and VAP episodes. There was one CAUTI event, giving a 60% reduction in CAUTI events between quarters. Some hidden cost containments were also obtained. Medication errors were reduced by 78%. The prevention of clinical errors and the avoidance of unnecessary blood draws are some examples. There was an improvement in the consistent messaging delivered to patients and their families and sign-outs between the day and night shift staff. The morale of the nursing staff also increased exponentially. As indicated in another case in this text, this active engagement model and other strategies helped to recruit and retain high-performing staff with specialized skills.

Conclusion

The interdisciplinary approach combined with the active engagement model has produced tangible and nontangible results in a short time. A strong partnership between various disciplines and departments is imperative to succeeding in quality measures within the hospital. We continue to refine the model by identifying unrecognized barriers and maximizing confidence and commitment among those involved in order to ensure continuous improvement in safety and quality for our patients and staff. One of the suggestions is to establish formal physician quality assurance directorship for the unit. Multiple initiatives have been introduced and are being reviewed. The 7 South ICU also created a new mission statement that will drive the future direction of quality care.

Conclusions

QUALITY MEASUREMENT FRAMEWORK

A framework that builds on the Institute of Medicine (IOM) definition of quality and integrates its six aims with the modified Donabedian framework of access, structure, process, outcome, and patient experience is described in this text. Although this framework has been applied (in the text) to the definition and measurement of quality of care in the inpatient hospital context, the principles apply to healthcare organizations in other contexts as well. The proposed framework can be implemented through the following general steps:

1. Define the healthcare context.
2. Define organizational operations; create related operational categories.
3. Link operational categories to the IOM aims.
4. Link operational measures to access, structure, process, outcome, and patient experience.
5. Link operational measures to the IOM aims.
6. Apply case-mix and other context-specific considerations.

A key feature of this framework is that it defines the organization's operations as a series of activities, each with a clear beginning and conclusion. As such, outcomes from one operation may be viewed as process measures for an operation that follows, and problems in one operation may be traced back to deficiencies in a preceding operation. Another significant feature of this framework is that it allows for the creation of indicators and metrics for each of the IOM aims at the level of an operation, categories of operations, or the organization overall. These measures, indicators, and metrics will also have a clearly defined relationship with the organization's access, structure, processes, outcomes, and patient experience domains, which will help in devising plans to improve quality of care.

This framework can be a useful addition to a performance measurement system in a healthcare organization in general and a hospital in particular.

FRAMEWORK FOR PERFORMANCE-DRIVEN PLANNING: INTEGRATION OF QUALITY AND FINANCE

As discussed throughout the text, quality improvement should not be considered only in terms of the initiatives and projects directed toward that operational objective. It should be thought of as a strategic asset and a powerful determinant of long-term viability of the organization. Quality performance is as important as financial performance; the two together are critical to the long-term viability and success of the organization. The use of a mission-based, performance-driven planning framework, one that allows constant monitoring of plan execution and real-time quality and financial results, is proposed as the optimal planning framework. At its core, in the context of a healthcare organization and specifically a hospital, it builds on the foundation of values and mission to establish financial and quality performance metrics. As financial performance has already been thoroughly addressed and developed, the focus of this text was placed on the quality dimension. In fact, the ideal managerial environment would be one where the control systems associated with quality performance were as fully developed and attended to as the financial systems.

Unlike financial performance, where the measures are currently more standardized, each organization will need to develop its own customized quality performance measures until such time as there is more meaningful standardization. Using the IOM definition of quality and the six aims underneath that definition, an organization can develop a customized system that measures what is most critical to the organization and also monitor the most relevant areas of quality depending on its patient-mix, types of procedures, and most common encounter type.

This recommendation is in contrast to a focus on generic Joint Commission measures. Although The Joint Commission (TJC) represents a significant pioneering and valuable effort in the field of quality, there is much more ground to be covered in healthcare quality than is currently addressed by TJC measures. For instance, with respect to TJC's core measures, one could point out the limited number of the diseases monitored: acute myocardial infarction, congestive heart failure, pneumonia, and surgical infections. Additionally, as stated earlier, it is not clear whether such things as prescribing of aspirin at discharge would necessarily translate into usage of aspirin by the patient. In fact, a hospital can implement mechanisms to ensure compliance with these measures, with barely noticeable changes in the overall quality of care delivered to its patients as measured by outcomes. This should not diminish the efforts by TJC; however, the time has come to think about quality of care in a more fundamental and strategic way. As a result, off-the-shelf quality measures may serve as a starting point for an organization, but they do not satisfy the need for a careful internal review of the access, structure process, and patient experience within the organization to identify comprehensive measures that encompass all functions of the organization and can be linked to outcomes. Once the *framework* for quality measures, indicators, and metrics within the organization is constructed, a careful study of financial performance consequences of positive and negative changes in that quality framework at different levels of measures, indicators, and metrics should be conducted. This will bring the organization to a point where it can fully evaluate and anticipate the consequences of strategic actions and proposals related to quality by providing management and governance with the necessary information to make complex and sometimes difficult decisions.

This same quality framework should maintain the balance between quality and finance by providing a sophisticated tool for monitoring quality of care and identifying points of intervention for corrective action. This ensures the consideration of both finance and quality in securing the overall long-term viability of the organization through the appropriate choice of strategy. Once a strategy is adopted and implementation begins, monitoring of performance will allow the organization to determine whether execution is proceeding according to plan. If the results are not consistent with expectations, remedies could be identified more readily by using the framework (by testing the hypotheses and selecting the best tactical move).

The quality performance data collected through the application of this framework will bring metrics to the performance dashboard and truly reflect the quality status of the organization. This should provide greater understanding to management and governance in exercising their responsibilities and in sharing the joint responsibility for the formulation of strategy.

Ultimately, the responsibility for ensuring an acceptable level of quality with respect to the care a healthcare organization provides lies with its board. It has been suggested that members should allocate at least 25% their meeting time to quality of care.[1] A customized dashboard is needed to provide the board with the tools and information it needs to monitor quality of care and set priorities for improving it at the organization.

For an organization to deliver high-quality care, the importance of quality must be communicated to all stakeholders. By use of values, mission, and vision statements and a clearly defined set of performance expectations, a message of quality could be presented in a comprehensive and meaningful way.

IMPLICATIONS AND LIMITATIONS OF THE FRAMEWORKS

As was discussed previously in this text, the field of quality in health care is younger and less mature than its counterparts in other industries; namely, manufacturing and service industries. Also, because of significant differences between the manufacturing and healthcare industries, some of the quality concepts in manufacturing are not readily transplanted into health care. Therefore, health care requires its own unique approach to quality that, while building on some concepts borrowed from manufacturing, can incorporate the peculiarities of health care into quality measurement for that industry.

Unfortunately, a consolidated approach to quality is still lacking in health care. Despite the multitude of organizations that are active in the field of health care quality, a consistent definition and measurement system cannot be found. The IOM definition is almost 20 years old[2] and has not been made operational in most (if not all) healthcare organizations. Other shortcomings include the limited list of measures, mostly process measures that encompass only a few limited clinical conditions. Finally, safety seems to be appropriately at the forefront of quality discussion. But, this seems to be at the expense of losing sight of the other five dimensions of quality as defined by the IOM.

The National Quality Forum (NQF) was created in 1998 to offer a forum for quality discussions and bring the stakeholders closer together. Perhaps a conversation at NQF is needed to refocus the healthcare quality agenda on a more comprehensive approach to quality such as the one presented in this text.

Quality measurements based on the framework presented in this text link quality to organizational operations. Therefore, the quality measurement framework provides a valuable tool for improvement of operations along the six aims introduced by the IOM. This has significant potential implications on organizational performance measurement and the organizational strategic planning process.

The main limitation of this framework and the multistep quality measurement system proposed here is that they have not been empirically studied. However, the conceptual framework presented in this text aims to provide a logical approach to the systematic and comprehensive measurement of quality in health care and as such would serve a constructive purpose in any healthcare organization.

AREAS FOR FUTURE RESEARCH

As stated in this text, the IOM definition of healthcare quality is explicit and comprehensive and should be adopted by all stakeholders. Even with the adoption of the IOM definition, current quality measures remain in relatively early stages of development and leave substantial room and need for future research. Today's health care clearly needs comprehensive and consistent quality measures capable of capturing the current level of quality and aiding the transition of healthcare quality to its next level.

In the end, whether the proposed framework in this text will allow healthcare organizations to integrate finance with quality and successfully improve the quality of care they deliver has to be empirically studied. As discussed in this text, current views of quality are very narrow, with significant emphasis on safety. The framework proposed here takes a logical approach to measurement and standardization of quality measures, indicators, and metrics and recognizes the full scope of quality. It also recognizes the critical role of quality in the organization's performance. How quickly these important concepts will be adopted by the healthcare industry and whether there will be any regulatory intervention remains to be seen.

This text focused on quality of care within a healthcare organization and the implications for quality and financial performance. It also examined the ways that quality performance can be integrated with the planning process. Finally, strategies that could lead to quality improvement were discussed.

However, it is naive to think that quality of care within a system such as the U.S. healthcare system can be improved by focusing only on quality within the delivery of care. Given the complexity of the U.S. healthcare system, a more comprehensive approach to all aspects of the healthcare system and implications for quality is needed. This is evident when one looks simply at the disappointing data on healthcare expenditures and outcomes in the United States compared with those of other industrialized countries.

U.S. healthcare expenditure per capita is more than that of other Organisation for Economic Co-operation and Development (OECD) countries,[3–6] and yet certain, important outcomes are worse.[7] What is becoming worrisome is that average spending on health per capita and total expenditure on health as percentage of gross domestic product (GDP) are growing at an accelerated pace in the United States compared with those in other industrialized nations,[8] although

Medicare spending growth may be slowing down.[9] No matter how one looks at it, projections show that the healthcare expenditures could grow to well over $3 trillion by 2015 even under the most conservative of assumptions.[8,10]

In such a complex environment, fixing one healthcare organization at a time cannot overhaul the entire system, mainly because there will not be any incentive for any single organization to endure the challenges associated with the substantial change that will be required. More research into all aspects of healthcare quality (and associated costs, if any) from a national perspective is needed. Access, which is one of five domains of care[11] and is related to equity of care, one of the six aims of quality as defined by IOM,[12] cannot be addressed from one organization's perspective and requires national initiatives and change in policy. Implications of recent changes at the national policy level were discussed previously in this text.

Another important area of research deals with the question of why the United States spends far more than other OECD countries per capita for health care. In 2007, total healthcare expenditure per capita in the United States was 50% more than that of the next most expensive OECD country and more than twice the average for OECD countries.[13] Spending per hospital visit is the highest in the United States, and U.S. life expectancy is among the bottom quartile among the OECD countries.[14] It is not hard to imagine that identifying and eliminating the causes of this wasteful spending produce a more efficient healthcare system. This, in turn, results either in more coverage for people at the same level of quality or improved quality outcome for the same level of expenditure.

Administrative costs (i.e., bureaucracy) makes up 30% to 31% of U.S. healthcare expenditure,[15,16] whereas in Canada, administration accounts for 16.7% of healthcare expenditure.[15] It is important to identify how much of this cost is dedicated to measuring and managing quality of care and whether any of it can be linked to improved outcomes.

The role of information technology and decision support systems is increasingly recognized as an important contributor to patient safety and quality of care. However, information technology is not exploited to its full potential, and further research, especially into decision support systems, is needed.

The significance of third-party payers must not be overlooked. When patients who receive care are unaware of the cost of care they receive because they are not financially responsible for the bill, they may not ask questions regarding less expensive alternatives to the medication that they receive or whether there is a less expensive test to diagnose their problem. At the same time, providers may have incentives to overuse the system. There is evidence that such attitudes may change when there is more financial responsibility for the patients or their families.[17,18] Also, there is evidence that consumer-directed health plans may result in lower costs,[19] but the full impact of this issue is not well understood and must be further studied.

Six Sigma is an attractive concept that has been implemented in manufacturing. It appears that healthcare organizations operate within two to four sigmas, which is far behind standards in other industries.[20] In some areas within a healthcare organization, it may be possible to close this gap; for example, errors during anesthesia or in processing of medication orders by the hospital pharmacy. This brings up the issue of input variation (patients). Again, this is an important fact of life in the practice of medicine, but its impact on the performance and quality of care is not fully understood. More research into creating models to determine the impact of input variation on output variation and adjustment for eliminating its effect is needed. Only then can points of diminishing returns be identified through nonempirical research and a more reasonable method for assessing the gap between the current defect rate and the Six Sigma ideal be estimated.

Finally, one should also recognize that the definition of quality and its dimensions—in the case of the IOM definition and its six aims—are not universally held and may be subject to significant variation in interpretation. Despite the fact that IOM's definition of quality is adopted here and its six aims are central to this text, one should be cognizant of the potential shortcomings of those aims. For example, patient centeredness is an aim. But what does it mean exactly? Is timeliness of care not a characteristic of patient-centered care? As can be seen here, these aims are not necessarily independent of one another and may not be at the same level in a hierarchical tree of quality priorities. Improvement in one dimension may result in improvement in performance in another dimension of quality as a result of this relationship. This an area that is not very well studied.

REFERENCES

1. Vaughn T, Koepke M, Kroch E, Lehrman W, Sinha S, Levey S. Engagement of leadership in quality improvement initiatives: executive quality improvement survey results. *J Patient Saf.* 2006;2(1):2–9.
2. Lohr KN. *Medicare: A Strategy for Quality Assurance.* Vol. 1. Washington, DC: Institute of Medicine; 1990.
3. *The US Healthcare System: Best in the World or Just the Most Expensive?* Orono, ME: The University of Maine; 2001.
4. Anderson GF, Frogner BK, Johns RA, Reinhardt UE. Health care spending and use of information technology in OECD countries. *Health Aff (Millwood.).* 2006;25(3): 819–831.

5. Anderson GF, Hussey PS, Frogner BK, Waters HR. Health spending in the United States and the rest of the industrialized world. *Health Aff (Millwood.)*. 2005;24(4): 903–914.

6. Anderson GF, Frogner BK, Reinhardt UE. Health spending in OECD countries in 2004: an update. *Health Aff (Millwood)*. 2007;26(5):1481–1489.

7. Rodwin VG. The health care system under French national health insurance: lessons for health reform in the United States. *Am J Public Health*. 2003;93(1):31–37.

8. Davis K, Schoen C, Guterman S, Shih T, Schoenbaum SC, Weinbaum I. Slowing the growth of U.S. health care expenditures: what are the options? In: *2007 Bipartisan Congressional Health Policy Conference*. Commonwealth Fund Pub. No. 989. New York, NY: The Commonwealth Fund; 2007.

9. White C. Why did Medicare spending growth slow down? *Health Affairs*. 2008; 27(3):793–802.

10. NHE summary including share of GDP, CY 1960-2010; Historical National Health Expenditure Data. Centers for Medicare & Medicaid Services website. http://www.cms.gov/Research-Statistics-Data-and-Systems/Statistics-Trends-and-Reports/National HealthExpendData/NationalHealthAccountsHistorical.html. Accessed April 9, 2012.

11. Domain framework and inclusion criteria. Agency for Healthcare Research and Quality website. http://www.qualitymeasures.ahrq.gov/about/domain-definitions .aspx. Accessed November 5, 2011.

12. Committee on Quality of Health Care in America. *Crossing the Quality Chasm: A New Health System for the 21st Century*. Washington, DC: Institute of Medicine; 2001.

13. OECD. Health expenditure per capita. In: *Health at a Glance 2009: OECD Indicators*. OECD Publishing; 2009.

14. Anderson GF, Squires DA. Measuring the U.S. health care system: a cross-national comparison. *Issue Brief (Commonw Fund)*. 2010;90:1–10.

15. Woolhandler S, Campbell T, Himmelstein DU. Costs of health care administration in the United States and Canada. *N Engl J Med*. 2003;349(8):768–775.

16. Blackstone EA, Fuhr Jr JP. Redefining health care: creating value-based competition on results. *Atlantic Economic Journal*. 2007;35(4):491–501.

17. Herrick DM. Update 2006: why are health costs rising? *Medical Benefits*. 2006; 23(20):6.

18. Chao LW, Pagan JA, Soldo BJ. End-of-life medical treatment choices: do survival chances and out-of-pocket costs matter? *Med Decis Making*. 2008;28(4):511–523.

19. Buntin MB, Damberg C, Haviland A, et al. Consumer-directed health care: early evidence about effects on cost and quality. *Health Affairs*. 2006;25:w516–w530.

20. Feazell GL, Marren JP. The quality-value proposition in health care. *J Health Care Finance*. 2003;30(2):1–29.

INDEX

Note: Italicized page locators indicate figures; tables are noted with *t*.

A

AAFP. *See* American Academy of Family Physicians

Abstraction, 107

Access, 54, 258

  calculating indicators for each operation, 126

  evaluating, 123

  Health Security Act and, 20

  NQMC domain and, 121

  old paradigm of, 180

  Patient Protection and Affordable Care Act and, 22

  performance-driven planning and, 181, *182*

  in U.S. healthcare system, 9, 11, 17–18

Access measures, operational measures linked to, 117–119, *118*

ACP. *See* American College of Physicians

Administrative costs, in U.S. *vs.* in Canada, 258

Adverse drug events, interruptions and cost of, 245

Adverse outcomes, organizational orientation and, 145–146

Adverse patient events

  litigation and, 66–67

  registered nurse staffing and lower risk of, 147

Advisory boards, 144

Advocacy organizations, in U.S. healthcare system, 4–5

Aesthetics, Garvin's dimension of, 63, 65

Affordable Health Care for America Act, 22

Agency for Healthcare Research and Quality, 21, 59, 84–85, 89, 93, 121, 167

Aging of population, healthcare cost containment and, 15

AHA. *See* American Hospital Association

AHCAA. *See* Affordable Health Care for America Act

AHIP. *See* America's Health Insurance Plans

AHQA. *See* American Health Quality Association

AHRQ. *See* Agency for Healthcare Research and Quality

AMA. *See* American Medical Association

Ambulatory Quality Alliance, 89–90

American Academy of Family Physicians, 89

American College of Physicians, 58, 89

American College of Surgeons

  Hospital Standardization Program of, 57

  National Surgical Quality Improvement Project, 200

American Health Quality Association, 90

American Hospital Association, 5, 58, 89

American Medical Association, 5, 58, 89

American Nurses Association, 5

American Recovery and Reinvestment Act of 2009, 23, 107, 147, 190